The Diabetes Diary

Dr. Gayle Eversole

By the same author

Blood Pressure Care Naturally

FOOD SAFETY: Cleansing Options

My Medicine Garden

My Happy Garden

The Garden Series

Health Matters

*herbal*YODA Says!

Wild Medicine

DEDICATION

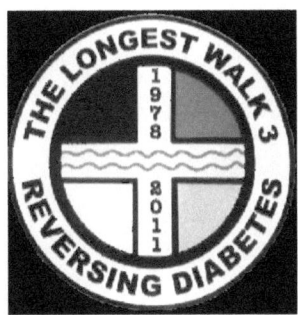

This book is dedicated to anyone anywhere that is affected directly or indirectly by diabetes, in what ever form it takes.

It is most importantly dedicated to my Native American sisters and brothers who have been struggling against the ravages of diabetes for far too many years.

CONTENTS

Acknowledgment   i

1   July   1

2   June   11

3   May   35

4   April   47

5   March   59

6   February   94

7   Diabetes Info &   105
    Tips

8   Diabetes E List   115

9   About CHI and   191
    the Author

ACKNOWLEDGMENT

Today is a Good Day for Walking -

Longest Walk 3, Reversing Diabetes: The Diabetes Diary

CHI supported this monumental event in the form of educational material about food and nutrition for diabetes, and related important information. This natural health education information is to help inform and to help prevent and reverse diabetes.

2011 National Diabetes Summit• July 05-07, 2011 • Washington, DC, USA - Washington DC will host the "Longest Walk 3" (Reversing Diabetes 2011) on July 8th, a 5000 mile walk/run relay across America to raise awareness of diabetes among Native Americans. The walkers left La Jolla (San Diego), California and Portland, Oregon on February 14 and walked and ran across the U.S.A. planning to arrive in Washington, DC on July 8, 2011.

Along the way the walkers have conducted forums on diabetes including juice fasts, exercising, walking, healthy diets and gardening at local tribal communities. They have visited over 40 American Indian reservations throughout the journey. The walk has provided the opportunity to collect diabetic concerns and stories from across America and to develop this information into a personal in-depth perspective from the Native view.

Activist Dennis Banks has spent most of his life fighting for Indian rights and now he's fighting a potentially bigger threat in Indian Country: diabetes.

Banks, 75, has been diagnosed with the disease. He has made major changes in his diet and lifestyle in order to lose weight and become more healthy.

"Food is medicine. We have to look at it that way," Banks said at the Yakama Healthy Heart Conference on the Yakama Nation. "We have to start viewing food as native people again."

Banks is one of the organizers of the Longest Walk 3. After visiting 54 reservations so far, he said as many as 50 percent of American Indians suffer from diabetes, with some reservations seeing a rate as high as 90 percent.

http://longestwalk3.com/ http://lw3.internettechnologyservice.net/

Historically the moving of our First People onto reservations and the forcing of non-traditional commodity foods made an in road to the development and rise of diabetes among the people. You often hear the story of the Pima people of the Southwest who have been decimated by this disease. The Pima are not alone.

Traditional foods have shown that they contribute greatly to the prevention and reversal of diabetes.

In the mid through late 1990s my organization provided a Diabetes Education Program on many western reservations based on many decades of commitment in natural health. We have been honored to be able to participate in the Longest Walk 3 in this small - but we hope beneficial - way.

CHI's website has a dedicated area for Diabetic Health. http://www.leaflady.org/Diabetic_Health.htm

CHI's blog has over 30 posts regarding health issues and diabetes. Here's the link, just use the search box to locate the articles: Natural Health News, http://naturalhealthnews.blogspot.com.

CHI publishes The Diabetes E List. This is an opt in subscription with a onetime $5 fee to join. The educational articles we have sent out are added at the end of the 'Diary". If you would like to subscribe please go to www.leaflady.org and send a $5 donation to CHI via our PayPal link and note Diabetes E List on your note in PayPal.

I hope in some small way this information serves as a guide to help you recover and heal. The guide is certainly incomplete but it represents all of the information made available in support of The Longest Walk. I hope even one small bit of this information is helpful to you.

Our little book, Blood Pressure Care Naturally, may be of interest to you if you have blood pressure problems. It is available here, www.createspace.com/3857772.

We publish *herbalYODA* Says! which is our free opt-in newsletter. You can subscribe at www.leaflady.org.

Throughout this document you will see the acronym *PWD. This stands for "People with Diabetes" and it is the choice we make to help defer from focusing on the disease rather than the people who live with it everyday.

I wish to extend my thanks to Evans Craig of the Navajo and Scot nations. Evans lives in the Washington DC area and served as National Coordinator for LW3. He is owner of Internet Technology Services, http://internettechnologyservice.net/

I am grateful for all of the new people I have met because of this event, and old friends with whom I have reconnected.

Christopher Francisco, Navaho, served as coordinator for the Northern Route which is the group closest to me geographically. Chris is based in Portland, Oregon.

I extend my thanks to Tracy Thomas, Mohawk, for his brilliant design of the Longest Walk III logo.

"The Ghost Walkers represent those who have walked before us...for our survival. Also to represent the walkers of 2011, who will walk in memory of relatives, who have passed from this devastating disease. To bring us hope for a change to a healthy lifestyle...The circle design is the four directions or the colors of humankind. The walk will have representation from the 4 directions, who will be taking part of this historic walk. Also pictured is the 3 sisters called; sustainers of life, this part of the circle...we call "Our Way of Life" Nyawenha/Thank you"

You can learn more about Chris and Terry at http://earthbornproductions.com/

Thank you to Chief Harry Goodwolf Kindness for allowing us to use his photo for the cover of this publication.

Thanks to all those who served as local and state coordinators who made this event even more amazing, all the walkers and supporters.

My thanks go as well to the efforts of Dennis Banks for keeping the dream alive.

It is good!

Remember, you can prevent and reverse diabetes!

1 JULY 2011

Water – Nature's almost perfect medicine. Pure water will help lower blood sugar by diluting the glucose levels in your blood. When you feel thirsty drink a glass of water. If your tongue feels like sandpaper then you know you are dehydrated. When you are dehydrated your health is at risk.

RESOURCES:

http://diabetesupdate.blogspot.com/2011/07/healthy-whole-grains-just-as-healthy-as.html

http://www.fathead-movie.com/index.php/2011/07/11/hope-warshaws-pepsi-challenge/

Some new reports for people with diabetes – Nutrition Research has found that a healthy diet can protect against excess oxidation. Expanding on those previous findings, a new study suggests that broccoli sprouts may be a star player for keeping oxidation in balance in people with type 2 diabetes. http://www.naturalproducts info.org/index.php?submenu=Health_Info&src=gendocs&r ef=Lookup&category=Lookup& resource=%2Fassets%2Ffeature %2Fbroccoli-sprouts-bolster-battle-against-type-2-diabetes_14271_4%2F%7Edefault

Grapes and Resveratrol - A plant chemical found in grapes and red wine known as resveratrol has become increasingly known for its heart health benefits. Now a new study in the British Journal of Nutrition suggests that resveratrol may also be good for blood sugar regulation. http://www.naturalproducts info.org/index.php? submenu=Health_Info&src=gendocs&ref=Lookup&category=Looku p& resource=%2Fassets%2Ffeature%2Fresveratrol-from-grapes-may-regulate-blood-suga r%2F%7Edefault

Hummus - from Chick peas to help your health, anti cancer too.

Hummus Recipe Ingredients: 1 can chickpeas - (15 oz), drained, reserving 1 tbsp of the liquid, 3 garlic cloves - (to 6), minced, 1 tbsp sesame tahini, Juice of 1 lemon, 2 tsp olive oil, 1 pinch cayenne pepper,

Recipe Instructions:

Combine all ingredients in a blender until smooth, using the 1 tablespoon chickpea liquid if necessary to make a smooth spread. This recipe yields 12 servings. Serving size: 2 tablespoons. Exchanges Per Serving: 1/2 Carbohydrate.

Nutrition Facts: Calories 49; Calories from Fat 17; Total Fat 2g; Saturated Fat 0g; Cholesterol 0mg; Sodium 33mg; Carbohydrate 7g; Dietary Fiber 2g; Sugars 1g; Protein 2g.

Diabetes medications alter nutrients for health

Diabetic Medications -

Includes sulfonylurea drugs such as Diabinese and Tolinase; second gener-ation drugs Glynase and Diabeta; and miscellaneous diabetes drugs such as Metformin and Acarbose.

Chromium: This mineral is essential for the body's metabolism of glucose. Low levels may lead to insulin insensitivity and abnormal insulin usage.

Vitamin C: Vitamin C improves all aspects of diabetes, and is often depleted because of free-radical destruction and increased urinary excretion.

Magnesium: There is a direct relation-ship between magnesium deficiency and insulin resistance. Magnesium also improves all aspects of diabetes aiding in arterial strength, normalizing blood pressure, and aiding in glycolysis. Most diabetics have an 80 to 85 percent deficiency.

Vitamins B6 and B12: B6 may aid in healthy eye support and proper vision.

Bilberry, lutein and other bioflavonoids may be supplemented when vision problems, diabetic retinopathy or macular degeneration are present. (Note: these herbs would be contraindicated with warfarin use or you can ask your doctor to lower the warfarin dose to compensate for the health benefit of these herbs.)

Folic Acid: Vitamin B9 or folate. A deficiency is especially noted with Metformin use as is vitamin B12.

Vitamin D supports balanced blood sugar levels and insulin sensitivity, according to a recently published study. Vitamin D is a fat-soluble vitamin ingested in the diet or made by the body upon exposure of the skin to sunlight. People with diabetes may need to take additional vitamin D beyond recommended levels to maintain blood status at 80 which allows for reserve and protection from depleted stores of this hormone like nutrient.

Carrots Help Lower Blood Sugar and make insulin work more effectively Carrots - Along with their many other health benefits, carotenoid-rich carrots may improve our ability to maintain healthy blood sugar levels. Research has suggested that dietary intake of carotenoids (and therefore higher blood levels of these beneficial compounds) may be inversely associated with insulin resistance and high blood sugar levels.

• Carrots with Honey Mustard Sauce

1 lb carrots, 1 tsp Dijon mustard, 2 tsp raw honey, 2 TBS extra virgin olive oil

Directions: Fill the bottom of the steamer with 2 inches of water. While steam is building up in steamer, cut carrots into 1/4-inch slices. Steam carrots for 5 minutes. Combine mustard, honey, and olive oil. Remove carrots from heat and toss with honey mustard mixture.

Serves 2 - http://whfoods.org/genpage .php?
tname=foodspice&dbid= 21

Carrots with mint is also yummy

Vinegar for your health, fights diabetes and many other things

Excellent for a hot weather drink - see *** Has magnesium which is
very good for people with diabetes, can keep many health problems
away. Make special herbal vinegars for specific health concerns. More
about vinegar at www.leaflady.org

• Vinegars in the kitchen? Pure health

All vinegars have significant health properties. Ancients had well
understood it, to the point of including them in their time
pharmacopeia. The list of popular remedies

by Luigi Caricato

http://www.luigicaricato.net/

Vinegars are healthy, provided that the raw material is of good quality,
because a vinegar ideally expresses its origin. It is necessary to well
work the product throughout its production, in order to keep its
substance content unaltered.

There are no doubts on vinegars nutritional and health value, as well as
for their preventive role for our health. It would be important to
acquire further information on this, and for this new researches are
expected. Here below, a list of indications which has been known since
the ancient times, popular remedies which are still important.

Vinegar:

- *** it is a thirst quenching drink, two spoons in a glass of water are
enough

- it is useful against stomachache, when feeling bloated, and against stomach

burning: one spoon in a glass of water is enough

- it is good against bad breath, for instance after waking up, it helps gargling

and swallowing two spoons of vinegar

- one spoon with sugar is effective against hiccups

- it is an excellent disinfectant on small wounds, because it attacks germs and

accelerates cicatrization (forming a scab)

- rubbing with pure vinegar acts against muscle and nerve numbness

- it is excellent against sore feet, with just two coffee cups in a foot bath

- it mitigates itching and burning sensations due to insect bites, just by applying it on the skin

- it has cosmetic functions, since it protects the skin from external agents and from an excessive use of alkaline soaps, restoring skin acidity- it makes hair brighter and restores hair pH, just with just one spoon while rinsing

- as an alternate option to anti lice shampoos, vinegar is the ideal solution, because it does not damage hair; a warm vinegar pack on wet hair for about half an hour solves the problem of lice, because acetic acid dissolves chitin through which lice stick nit to the hair

04 July 2011 Teatro Naturale International n. 7 Year 3

Coconut oil, a healthy fat for people with diabetes

Some people will use a teaspoon of coconut oil before meals to prevent heartburn. Some people use coconut oil to resolve symptoms of GERD (acid reflux).

• Some people use it to combat heat rash and fungal infections, especially under skin folds.

• Massage into your scalp to nourish hair and clear scalp problems.

"Why is Coconut Oil so good for you and how does it help burn fat?"

Coconut oil is made up of medium-chain fatty acids (MCFA's) which are a great aid in losing weight, lowering cholesterol, and reducing the risk of cardiovascular disease. MCFA's will give you immediate energy and increased thermogenesis (fat burning) which also helps circulation. MCFA's do not require the liver and gallbladder to digest and emulsify them. If your digestion is compromised or you have had your gallbladder removed, coconut oil is the only oil you should use as it is very easily digested. Coconut oil is also helpful for those with underactive thyroid, common in people with diabetes (also fatty liver, gall bladder problems and wheat allergy, more).

Fiber is very important for PWD as it helps maintain lower blood sugar levels.

There are two main types of fat in our bodies: subcutaneous and visceral. Subcutaneous is the fat right under the skin, which is more visible but does not pose as much of a health threat as visceral fat.

Visceral fat, or "belly fat," can be found surrounding our organs. Ailments caused by high levels of this type of fat include high blood pressure, diabetes, liver disease...the list goes on and on.

There have been many studies on the positive effects of fiber and how it can fight fat in the body.

However, few studies of fat and fiber have focused on specific types of fiber and their effects on specific types of body fat.

A new study from Wake Forest Baptist Medical Center in Winston-Salem, NC, offers strong evidence that eating soluble fiber (that is, fiber from vegetables, fruit, and beans), along with getting moderate exercise, can reduce harmful visceral fat in the body. Researchers compared body scans and self reported eating and exercise habits of more than 1,000 people, and found that for every 10 grams of fiber reported in their daily diet, visceral fat was about 3.7 percent lower. Subjects who reported engaging in moderate exercise (30 minute of vigorous activity two to four times a week) had even lower levels of visceral fat.

Even small changes you make in your diet have the potential to make a big impact on your overall health. Eating 10 grams of fiber more a day is easily attainable; in fact you can get just about 10 grams by eating any of these foods in these amounts:

• 2 apples

• ½ cup of pinto beans

• 1¼ cups of raspberries

• 1 cup of bran flakes

• 1 cup of vegetarian baked beans

• 1 artichoke

• 2 cups of broccoli

Other high fiber-foods include: carrots, brown rice, strawberries, oatmeal, lima and black beans, almonds, peas, sweet corn

Aminosweet is the new name for aspartame to fool you. Avoid this as with all other chemically based artificial sweeteners. They are known to cause diabetes.

Neotame – A more highly concentrated from of aspartame - Neotame is the technical name for a new sweetener developed by Monsanto Chemical Corp. It is reported to be approximately 8,000 times sweeter than sugar. The chemical formula for neotame was published in the February 10, 1998 Federal Register. It is quite similar in structure to Monsanto's toxic sweetener aspartame. There have not been any legitimate, independent, long-term human studies on neotame. Much sweeter than aspartame and much more toxic. These chemical sweeteners alter your taste buds so you lose your ability to taste "sweet" normally.

IV therapy for diabetes used to improve glucose metabolism, improve neuropathy, and vascular disease associated with diabetes. IV nutrients including alpha lipoic acid, folic acid, b12, thiamin, and ubichinon compositum, etc. IV Nutritional Therapies http://vitamincoach.com Intravenous IV Therapies performed at Medical Wellness Associates, Jeannette, PA.

Supplements Helpful for Fatty Liver - The following supplements have been shown to boost liver health and help manage NAFLD:

Vitamin E—800 IU daily includes at least 200 mg gamma tochopherol.

Omega-3 fatty acids—700 mg EPA and 500 mg DHA daily

S-adenosylmethionine (SAMe)—1200 mg daily

N-acetyl cysteine (NAC)—1200 mg daily

Silymarin (milk thistle extract)—900 mg daily

Polyenylphosphatidylcholine (PPC)—900 mg daily

Trans-resveratrol—500 mg daily

Other studies used Metformin—500 mg three times daily but his can be risky if you do not have diabetes. Metformin causes B12 to be destroyed. This research supports old data about diabetes and fat digestion problems, and why we suggest Milk Thistle (Silymarin) to help protect and nourish your liver with FLD and diabetes especially, much better than statins!

Another Cholesterol Myth The effect drugs (or anything else) have on cholesterol is irrelevant – it's the impact they have on health that counts. Read more http://www.drbriffa.com/2011/06/29/how-todesign-a-trial-to-ensure-you-dont-get-the-result-you-dont-want/

2 JUNE 2011

Diabetes, Pollution and Drugs: Another in support of what we've been stating for a long time.

[1]
http://www.isletsofhope.com/diabetes/complications/amputation_1.html

[2] Strong Link Between Diabetes and Air Pollution Found in National U.S.

Study.
http://www.sciencedaily.com/releases/2010/09/100929105654.htm

[3] ROS (Reactive Oxygen Species) are natural byproducts of oxygen metabolism in the body. Free radicals and other byproducts are formed as a result of this metabolism, and at lower levels can be very beneficial, but when too many of these byproducts are formed the situation of oxidative stress occurs. reactive oxygen species (ROS) include oxygen ions, free radicals and peroxides both inorganic and organic. They are generally very small molecules and are highly reactive due to the presence of unpaired valence shell electrons. Oxidative stress is a medical term for damage to animal or plant cells (and thereby the organs and tissues composed of those cells) caused by excesses of these reactive oxygen species, which include (but are not limited to) superoxide, singlet oxygen, peroxynitrite or hydrogen peroxide. Superoxide is produced deleteriously by 1-electron transfers in the mitochondrial electron transfer chain. It is defined as an imbalance between pro-oxidants and anti-oxidants, with the former prevailing. The causes of these excesses are many, and include environmental influences of every type. Enzyme activities are sometimes affected negatively, leading to greater production of excess ROS, and heavy metals such as chromium, vanadium, and others are said to be involved, now this new evidence that methylmercury definitely plays a

significant role in the pancreas. Cells are normally able to defend themselves against ROS damage through the use of enzymes such as superoxide dismutases and catalases. Small molecule antioxidants such as Ascorbic acid (vitaminC), uric acid, and glutathione also play important roles as cellular antioxidants. Similarly, Polyphenol antioxidants assist in preventing ROS damage by scavenging free radicals. Studies are conflicting on some antioxidants such as Vit. E. The resulting inflammatory processes are believed to be the result of these ROS excesses and include cardiovascular disease, ALS, neurodegenerative diseases, and many others.

[4] Kajimoto, Y., and Kaneto, H. (2004) Role of oxidative stress in pancreatic beta-cell dysfunction. Ann. N. Y. Acad. Sci. 1011, 168-176.

[5] Tiedge, M., Lortz, S., Drinkgern, J., and Lenzen, S. (1997) Relation between antioxidant enzyme gene expression and antioxidative defense status of insulin-producing cells. Diabetes 46, 1733-1742.

[6] Inoue, M., Sato, E. F., Nishikawa, M., Hiramoto, K., Kashiwagi, A., and Utsumi, K. (2004) Free radical theory of apoptosis and metamorphosis. Redox Rep. 9, 237-247.

[7] Rolo, A. P., and Palmeira, C. M. (2006) Diabetes and mitochondrial function: Role of hyperglycemia and oxidative stress. Toxicol. Appl. Pharmacol. 212, 167-178.

[8] American Chemical Society (2006, September 29). Mercury Compound Found In Fish Damages Pancreatic Cells. ScienceDaily. Retrieved June 27, 2011
http://www.sciencedaily.com/releases/2006/09/060925114107.htm

[9] Most of today's pharmaceutical preparations, because of their harmful effects, may be labeled poisonous," says chemist Dr Lisa Landymore-Lim, who has worked for the National Institute for Medical Research, London, and the Dunn Nutrition Unit, Cambridge. Her 1994 book, Poisonous Prescriptions, describes Landymore-Lim's investigations which have found that diabetes may in fact be a major

side effect of antibiotics and other common pharmaceuticals. The book provides evidence from studies and hospital records. Diabetes, usually thought to be largely a genetic disorder, may actually have increased so much in the last 50 years because of the proliferation in the use, and over-use, of medicines.

Drugmakers angle for advantage in treating diabetes Money more important than health http://news.yahoo.com/drugmakers-angle-advantage-treating-diabetes-155016341.html

Fiber-Up drinks are now available from Just Like Sugar, and safe sugar substitute too made from all natural ingredients. justlikesugarinc.com

Fat mediation needs your consideration Fat cells play key role in development of type 2 diabetes

www.sciencedaily.com Cellular changes in fat tissue -- not the immune system -- lead to the "hyperinflammation" characteristic of obesity-related glucose intolerance and type 2 diabetes, according to new research.

http://www.ncbi.nlm.nih.gov/pmc/articles/PMC3010636/ more on related issues

Related study
http://www.nutraingredients.com/content/view/print/382937

Merck using PR to cause fear and push drug sales New Survey Reveals Gap in Understanding of the Risk of Cardiovascular Disease for People with Type 2 multivu.prnewswire.com More Than One-third of Type 2 Diabetes Patients Over the Age of 40 State That They Are Not Receiving Cholesterol-Lowering Treatment

There are proven natural therapies to prevent and reverse cardiovascular dis-ease and lower LDL cholesterol, raise HDL cholesterol.

Bladder cancer risks aren't likely to stop sales of the diabetes drug pioglitazone (Actos) Medical News:

ADA: FDA Unlikely to Zap Pioglitazone - in Meeting Coverage, ADA from MedPage Today

www.medpagetoday.com SAN DIEGO -- Bladder cancer risks aren't likely to send the diabetes drug pioglitazone (Actos) down the same path as rosiglitazone (Avandia), according to this exclusive InFocus report from the ADA.

Why it is important to use your options to prevent, reduce and eliminate diabetes.

Explain that the antipsychotic drugs ripiprazole (Abilify), olanzapine (Zyprexa), and risperidone

(Risperdal) appear to increase body fat and risk of metabolic abnormalities in children and adolescents. Medical News: ADA: Antipsychotics Change Metabolism in Kids - in Meeting Coverage, ADA from MedPage. www.medpagetoday.com SAN DIEGO -- Antipsychotics appear to increase body fat and increase the risk of metabolic abnormalities in children and adolescents, researchers said here.

More - **Diabetes from fluoride based and Genetically Engineered (GE) drugs.**

Holy basil is used in some people with diabetes to decrease their blood sugar levels. Preliminary evidence has shown that holy basil leaf extract may decrease both fasting blood glucose levels and blood glucose after meals in type 2 diabetics.

'MyPlate' Food Makeovers 8 'MyPlate' Food Makeovers - Diet & Nutrition Center - Everyday Health www.everydayhealth.com Here's how to make your family's favorite meals fit the latest MyPlate food icon, which replaces the old food pyramid as part of the government's healthy eating food guidelines.

Satisfy Your Appetite With These Delicious Choices The 10 Most Filling Foods - Digestive Health Center - Everyday Health www.everydayhealth.com The most filling foods offer healthy volume without loading you up with empty calories. Include these healthy foods to manage weight and feel full longer.

27 Ways Herbs Add Instant Flavor to Recipes

27 Ways Herbs Add Instant Flavor to Recipes www.kitchendaily.com

Intensive dietary counseling helps improve glycemic control Medical News: ADA: Regular Diet Counseling Aids Glycemic Control - in Meeting Coverage, ADA from Med Page www.medpagetoday.com

SAN DIEGO -- Intensive dietary counseling in the year following a diagnosis of diabetes improved glycemic control, but adding exercise to the mix didn't add any extra benefits, researchers said here.

This is the very basis of nutritional education for prevention and reversal of this condition. Or any health condition for that matter! Too often doctors just give pills or insulin first and overlook the importance of nutrition and how it can reverse diabetes.

Why sleepiness is not always caused by a lack of sleep, diabetes Why sleepiness is not always caused by a lack of sleep | Dr Briffa's Blog - A Good Look at Good Health www.drbriffa.com I came across this story earlier this week. It concerns a study presented at a Associated Professional Sleep Societies in Minneapolis in the US. The details are...

Is Type 1 Diabetes Being Ignored? - Diabetes Center – Everyday Health www.everydayhealth.com Type 1 and type 2 diabetes are very different. Some people believe their names should be less similar to encourage more funding for type 1, but others disagree.

Vitamin D3 and Zinc are very important for people with Type 1. Hepatitis vaccine is a direct link to Type 1, guess why Type 1 rates are rising....

Old good news - vitamin E Health Promotion and Disease Prevention www.leaflady.org Why would you need statin drugs with these scientifically proven uses for vitamin E, C, all antioxidants? Using antioxidants is one of the most effective means of bringing about the regression and/or disappearance of cancer, according to a study done at Harvard's School of Dental Medicine.

Vitamin E is a first line defense against cancer by enhancing immunity, fighting free radicals, and preventing the formation of carcinogens in the intestine. (Tufts U. study)

Protein glycosylation in diabetics is prevented and triglyceride levels are lowered because of vitamin E of at least 100 IU daily. Orthomolecular medicine studies show that this needs to be 1600 IU daily.

U. Texas SW Medical Center showed that 800 IU vitamin E daily for 3 months showed reduction of LDL oxidation by 40 percent. Arterial blockage has shown to be reduced up to 60 percent in two years with vitamin E at 108 IU daily.

Harvard showed that vitamin E of 100 IU daily reduced heart dis-ease by 37 percent. The World Health Organization showed that vitamin E was more likely to prevent fatal heart attacks than lowering cholesterol.

The prevalence of diabetic kidney disease in the U.S. population has risen in parallel with the rates of diabetes, researchers said. NOTE: Many newer drugs for diabetes are genetically engineered. These drugs have a side effect of kidney failure. Artificial sweeteners also contribute to worsening diabetes and kidney problems. Poor nutrition & dietary advice from The Plate and Pyramid contribute to this.

Medical News: Diabetic Kidney Disease on Rise - in Nephrology, General Nephrology from MedPage Today www.medpagetoday.com

The prevalence of diabetic kidney disease has risen in parallel with rates of diabetes in the U.S., researchers said.

High-dose statins increase the risk of diabetes, another report High-dose statins increase the risk of diabetes...very slightly, study says www.latimes.com Intensive therapy with cholesterol-lowering statins increases the risk of developing diabetes slightly, but reduces the risk of cardiovascular disease more, Scottish researchers reported Tuesday. High doses of the drugs can increase the risk of developing Type 2 diabetes by about 12%...

You can lower cholesterol levels with good thyroid support, foods, and supplements.

Nerve Health Enhanced with Vitamins and Minerals

Salt, the beneficial kind Celtic salt, the CHI recommended salt for health. Celtic Sea Salt® Brand Sea Salts contain a higher percentage of mineral-dense natural brine (sea water). This bio-available high moisture content naturally lowers the amount of Sodium Chloride found in our salts. Hand-harvested, unrefined Celtic Sea Salt® Brand Sea Salts are recommended by Doctors and Natural Health Practitioners around the world. Both salt types from Grain & Salt Society are 23% and 17 % mineral base compared to 4% in toxic Himalayan salt.

Garlic lowers cholesterol, fights nail fungus.

Torshi is a traditional Persian pickled vegetable recipe. I can be made with any single or mixed vegetables. I have some garlic torshi brewing right now and it is very easy to make. Often in the US we ignore sour and bitter foods which actually are the best for digestive health. Using a glass jar with a plastic lid (don't use metal because the vinegar will react with it) peel the garlic cloves and place in jar. Fill with white wine vinegar vinegar , cover and let "pickle" for a week or two, then you have it. Eat with meals. I sometimes use as blend of white wine and rice vinegar Wikipedia says "Torshi (Arabic:

Turshi, Persian: torshi, Turkish: tursu, Greek: \]^_`a

toursi, Bulgarian: bcdefg turshiya, Bosnian: turšija) refers to pickled vegetables in the cuisine of many Balkan and Middle East countries. The word torshi comes from the Persian word torsh, which means 'sour'.

Tursu is common in Persian, Afghan, Turkish, Middle Eastern cuisine, Albanian, Armenian, Greek, Bulgarian, Macedonian, Serbian, and Bosnian. Iran boasts a great variation of hundreds of different types of torshi according to regional customs and different events. In some families, no meal is considered complete without a bowl of torshi on the table. In Bulgarian cuisine the most popular types are tsarska turshiya 'king's pickle' and selska turshiya 'country pickle'. Toursi is a traditional appetizer (meze) to go with rakı, ouzo, tsipouro, and rakia.

Making tursu at home is still a widespread tradition during the autumn months, even in the big cities.

Tursu is often served in restaurants or it can be bought prepared from large supermarkets."

see http://www.iranchamber.com/recipes/recipes.php

It's your thyroid and doctor's either ignore this or do not know! I found this on everyday health and was sort of surprised I did. Do not draw the conclusion you need cholesterol lowering drugs if your thyroid is not functioning properly. Problem is that docs refuse to order the proper thyroid panel of tests and the vast majority cannot interpret the results. Triglycerides when elevated will kill you, cholesterol has nothing to do with anything but make $$$ for Big PhRMA. I edited a little bit.

"More than 100 million American adults have elevated cholesterol, and no two cases are exactly alike.

While many people have high cholesterol because to poor diet, a sedentary lifestyle, lack of exercise, or simply because of heredity, other health conditions can put you at risk — especially conditions that affect the body's metabolism.

"When we see people who come in for assessment of an elevated form of LDL cholesterol or triglycerides, we always want to look for associated metabolic abnormalities," says Stephen J. Nicholls, MBBS, PhD, clinical director of the Cleveland Clinic Center for Cardiovascular Diagnostics and Prevention. These often include conditions like diabetes and hypothyroidism, an underactive thyroid.

High Cholesterol: Health Conditions That Put You at Risk

There are a number of health conditions that can lead to high cholesterol levels, and people who have them need to understand that they're at risk. Since high cholesterol is a major risk factor for heart disease, keeping it under control is essential. Knowing your risk is the first step to prevention.

Health conditions are known to increase cholesterol levels:

Diabetes (insufficient production of the hormone insulin)

Obesity/overweight

Kidney disease

Cushing's syndrome (an excess production of hormones)

Hypothyroidism (another hormonal imbalance)

Liver diseases like cirrhosis and nonalcoholic steatohepatitis

Alcoholism

There are a few reasons why these health conditions raise cholesterol levels. First, the levels of cholesterol and triglycerides in the blood "essentially reflect how our body works to metabolize the fat and cholesterol that we eat in a day," says Nicholls. "I think that diabetes and thyroid disorders can affect the way we metabolize cholesterol and triglycerides." This has a direct effect on triglyceride and cholesterol levels, he says. So when these conditions begin affecting metabolism and slowing it down, the body isn't able to process everything it needs to, including cholesterol.

Cholesterol drugs are known to cause KIDNEY FAILURE and muscle wasting.

New studies show supplements help lower blood sugar and eliminate neuropathy just like I have been stating for decades.

Chromium Supplementation and Glycemic Control

Keywords: DIABETES MELLITUS TYPE 2, GLYCEMIC CONTROL - Chromium

Reference:"Beneficial effect of chromium supplementation on glucose, HbA(1)C and lipid variables in individuals with newly onset type-2 diabetes," Sharma S, Agrawal RP, et al, J Trace Elem Med Biol, 2011

May 11; [Epub ahead of print]. (Address: College of Home Science, MPUA&T, Udaipur, Rajasthan, India).

Summary: In a placebo-controlled, single-blinded, prospective study involving 40 newly onset type 2 diabetics, daily supplementation with chromium (9 g brewer's yeast containing 42 microg chromium) for a period of 3 months was found to be associated with significant reductions in fasting blood glucose levels (197.65 to 103.68 mg/dL) and improvements in HbA(1)c (from 9.51 to 6.86), suggesting improved glycemic control. In addition, improvements in total cholesterol (from 199 to 189 mg/dL), triglycerides (from 144.94 to 126.01), and LDL cholesterol levels (from 119.19 to 99.58) were found. The authors state, "These data demonstrate beneficial effect of chromium supplementation on glycaemic control and lipid variables in subjects with newly onset type-2 diabetes."

GTF Chromium has been used for decades to help with blood sugar concerns.

FDA Warns of Bladder Cancer Risk With Actos - WASHINGTON -- Patients taking pioglitazone (Actos) for more than a year may have an increased risk of bladder cancer, according to an FDA review of interim data from an ongoing study. The update to the drug's warning label comes days after two European countries banned use of the drug.

Watching TV Ups Risk for Diabetes

Greek Yoghurt for People with Diabetes Greek yoghurt is just regular plain yoghurt that has been strained overnight in a yoghurt strainer to make it thinker. The whey that is removed is very healthy too.

So you see you can make your own. "Greek yogurt also has more protein and fewer carbs than traditional yogurt. This means that Greek yogurt can be appropriate for people with diabetes, says Tami Ross, RD, LD, a diabetes educator and vice-president of the American Association of Diabetes Educators.

"My patients love the consistency of it," explains Ross. "Even the patients who are not big on yogurt or milk products overwhelmingly seem to like Greek yogurt."

Greek yogurt's thick consistency comes from straining it to remove liquid whey. This process increases the amount of protein per serving and removes some of the carbohydrates, which people with diabetes must watch carefully.

"For folks with diabetes, the lower carbs are a plus," Ross notes. "You can work in the yogurt for a snack without having to account for so many carbohydrates."

The increased protein can also help you feel that you've had a more substantial snack, so you'll feel more satisfied and won't be hungry for something else quite so quickly. "In terms of promoting satiety and helping people feel full, it's great," Ross says. "

Cabbage and a note on vitamin C

Get radiation out of your water and related stories

Powerhouse

Blood Sugar Benefits from Summer Squash - The list of nutrients in summer squash related to healthy blood sugar regulation is a long one. Metabolism of sugar in the body requires ample presence of many B- complex vitamins, and most of these B-complex vitamins are found in valuable amounts in summer squash. Included here are the B-vitamins folate, B6, B1, B2, B3, and choline. Also important in blood sugar metabolism are the minerals zinc and magnesium, as well as omega-3 fatty acids, and all of these nutrients are provided by summer squash.

A mainstay of dietary protection from type 2 diabetes - as well as a key step in food support of diabetes problems - is optimal intake of fiber. Summer squash not only provides a very good amount of dietary fiber at 2.5 grams per cup, but it also provides polysaccharide fibers like pectin that have special benefits for blood sugar regulation. The pectin polysaccharides in summer squash often include chains of D-galacturonic acid called homogalacturonan. An increasing number of animal studies now show that these components in summer squash help keep insulin metabolism and blood sugar levels in balance, and protect against the onset of type 2 diabetes. For more   information see whfoods.org

The benefit of Coconut oil - Improves insulin secretion and utilization of blood glucose. Coconut Research Center www.coconutresearchcenter.org Your source for accurate information on the health and nutritional aspects of coconut, coconut oil, palm, palm oil, and related subjects. The scientific name for coconut is Cocos nucifera. Early Spanish explorers called it coco, which means "monkey face" because the three indentations (eyes) on the shell.

More Bad Results on the Cholesterol Drug Front Cholesterol-reducing drug ezetimibe appears to do more harm than good Cholesterol is said to cause heart disease (I'm not so sure, myself), and a mainstay of treatment here is a class of drugs known as 'statins' that reduce the rate at which cholesterol is manufactured in the liver. Statins have been used in medicine for over 20 years, but more recently has seen the development and licensing of a cholesterol-reducing drug known as ezetimibe, which works in different way to statins. Instead of acting on the liver, it reduces cholesterol absorption from the gut.

There's no doubt that ezetimibe reduces cholesterol levels effectively, and it is licensed on this basis.

However, the impact that a drug (or food or anything) has on cholesterol is irrelevant – it's its impact on health that matters. While we have been brainwashed into believing that whatever reduces cholesterol is good for health, this simply isn't true. Actually, there is abundant evidence that reducing cholesterol per se is not broadly beneficial to health. And some evidence suggests that it might even be damaging to health.

As it happens, ezetimibe use has been linked with an increased risk of cancer, and enhanced narrowing of arteries (though not statistically significant) [1], as well as an increased risk of cancer in one study [2].

Ezetimibe is a drug that reduces cholesterol levels in the bloodstream. It does this in a different way to statins (the most commonly-prescribed cholesterol drugs). Statins work by inhibiting the rate at which cholesterol is manufactured in the liver, while ezetimibe impairs the absorption of cholesterol from the gut.

Ezetimibe was originally licensed on the basis of its cholesterol-reducing abilities. Yet, to date, no study has ever been published which demonstrates that it has the power to reduce the risk of actual disease or death. In fact, in one study, coupling ezetimibe with a statin (simvastatin) resulted in increased (though not statistically significant) narrowing of the arteries compared to the statin alone [1].

I was interested to read a recent study in which ezetimibe was again tested for its affects on narrowing in the arteries (atherosclerosis) [3]. In this study, individuals with 'peripheral vascular disease' (atherosclerosis in the arteries in the legs) had the extent of their disease measured using MRI. Here's how the individuals in the study were treated:

1. those not previously on a statin were given simvastatin (40 mg a day) or simvastatin (40 mg a day) plus ezetimibe (10 mg a day).

2. those already taking a statin had ezetimibe (10 mg a day) added to their regime.

MRI was repeated after 1 and 2 years. Here's what the results showed:

Overall, ezetimibe resulted in lower 'unhealthy' LDL-cholesterol levels when used in conjunction with the statin than the statin alone. However, individuals in group 2 saw a progression of their disease (by 8 per cent over two years), compared with no progression in group 1.

In other words, in those taking a statin, the addition of ezetimibe actually worsened their disease.

This study, on the back of previous evidence, strongly suggests that ezetimibe poses hazards for health.

Yet, it remains on the market. This is what can happen when our attention is diverted away from the truly important thing (health), towards cholesterol or some other supposed marker of disease.

References:

1. Kastelein JJ, et al. Simvastatin with or without ezetimibe in familial hypercholesterolemia. NEJM 2008;358(14):1431-43

2. Rossebø AB, et al. Intensive Lipid Lowering with Simvastatin and Ezetimibe in Aortic Stenosis. NEJM 2008;359(13):1343-56

3. West AM, et al. The effect of ezetimibe on peripheral arterial atherosclerosis depends upon statin use at baseline. Atherosclerosis. 2011 Apr 16. [Epub ahead of print]

URL to article: http://www.drbriffa.com/2011/06/10/cholesterol-reducing-drug-ezetimibe-appears-todo-more-harm-than-good/

Cancer Risk Forces Actos Off French, German Markets

By John Gever, Senior Editor, MedPage Today, June 10, 2011

Drug regulators in Germany and France have ordered doctors to stop prescribing the type 2 diabetes drug pioglitazone (Actos) following a French study suggesting a heightened risk of bladder cancer.

The Importance of Protein I do not recommend soy unless it is in a fermented form such as tempeh. Soy has too many downside risks and it can be harmful to your thyroid. Avoid Glucerna because it is a commercially processed product even though promoted by ADA.

Longest Walkers - be very careful because of the high heat and humidity. Drink a lot of fluids for sure!

Water helps reduce blood sugar in the blood. We like Aquasana filters.

The Diabetes Assist Dog Diabetes Dog – iVillage www.ivillage.com For those who get a dog trained to assist diabetes patients, it can be mean life or death.

Turmeric helpful for neuropathy Turmeric Supplementation in Individuals with Type 2 Diabetic

Neuropathy

Keywords:DIABETES TYPE 2, END-STAGE RENAL DISEASE, DIABETIC NEUROPATHY - Turmeric, Curcumin

Reference: "Oral supplementation of turmeric attenuates proteinuria, transforming growth factor-beta and interleukin-8 levels in patients with overt type 2 diabetic nephropathy: A randomized, double-blind and placebo-controlled study," Khajehdehi P, Pakfetrat M, et al, Scand J Urol Nephrol, 2011 May 31;

[Epub ahead of print]. (Address: P. Khajehdehi, Department of Medicine, Nephro-Urology Research Center, Shahid Faghihi Hospital, Shiraz University of Medical Sciences, Shiraz, Iran. E-mail: khajehdp@hotmail.com).

Summary: In a randomized, double-blind, placebo-controlled study involving 40 patients with overt type 2 diabetic nephropathy, supplementation with turmeric (500 mg per capsule, each containing 22.1 mg curcumin, taken 3 times/day, with each meal), for a period of 2 months, was found to be associated with significant decreases in TGF-beta and IL-8 and urinary protein excretion, suggesting that, "Short-term turmeric supplementation can attenuate proteinuria, TGF-beta and IL-8 in patients with overt type 2 diabetic nephropathy and can be administered as a safe adjuvant therapy for these patients."

A Basic Health Action to Benefit Your Digestion and GI System from my colleague and longtime friend.

THE MORNING COOL-WATER G.I. TRACT REVIVER

Dr. Bruce Berkowsky's 21st Century Natural Health Science www.naturalhealthscience.com

Bruce Berkowsky, N.M.D., M.H., H.M.C. Copyright 2011 by Joseph Ben Hil-Meyer Research, Inc.

INTRODUCTION Due to modern man's propensity for eating highly processed foods.

Very helpful for hydration which is so important. My mother always did this.

Nutrition Research for Diabetes

There are people who just understand the basics of cellular medicine, and act appropriately. Dr. John Young in Tampa Florida has been experimenting with a new process for reversing metabolic syndrome and Type 2 diabetes over the past seven years, and claims to have a success rate of 80 percent with over 100 diabetes patients. Dr. Young uses a combination of alkaline protein and minerals with a form of iodine that he says reverses the process in diabetes patients in eight to 12 weeks. For those afflicted with Type 2 diabetes, his solution resets the pancreas and permanently returns patients to normal. Dr. Young has had success with pre-diabetes patients, who have blood sugar levels from 100 to 125, and Type 2 patients, who have blood sugar levels much higher.

http://www.depauw.edu/news/index.asp?id=22117

Myer's Cocktail - V vitamin and mineral therapy developed in the 1970's by John Meyer, M.D., a physician at Johns Hopkins University. The "cocktail" is indicated for chronic fatigue, Fibromyalgia, Depression, muscle spasm, Asthma, hives, Congestive Heart Failure, Angina(chest pain), infections, and Senile Dementia.

Dr. Glenn Rothfield has a website response that I will forward to you due to time constraints. I always used the most affordable ingredients, and did not use Glutathione. I feel that NAC (N-Acetyl Cysteineoral) gives so much value for the money that the need for glutathione can be met for days with this oral product; however, there is magic in giving safe nutrients rather rapidly. Magnesium and B complex are the MINIMUM in this cocktail with other ingredients based on the patient's needs. We used to have Adrenal Cortex and this was great and the glycyrrhizin when obtained from the right source is VERY useful.

The idea is that CALCIUM EDTA opens up a new world in which we can give almost anything with it or before it, from lots of IV Vitamin C to simply putting it in a mini bottle of 50 cc with some B complex and magnesium and let it drip for 5-30 minutes. We can amplify most of the chelation benefits without the time or pain involved previously. IV nutrition really is amazing as no matter how many vitamins and minerals we swallow, when given in a short time intravenously MOST patients SEE and FEEL a difference.

Sincerely,

Garry F. Gordon, MD,DO,MD(H)

Myers Cocktail by Glenn Rothfeld M.D.

Hundreds of physicians around the U.S. use this therapy, which is largely unknown and not much written about. The Myers Cocktail is named for the late John Myers, M.D., a Maryland physician who used intravenous injections of nutrients to treat his patients. Currently, the nutrient cocktail has been popularized by Alan Gaby, M.D., president of the American Holistic Medical Association and a physician who writes a lot about nutritional factors in medicine.

The idea of the Myers Cocktail is that many illnesses and conditions are associated with digestive disturbances such as bloating, maldigestion and food sensitivities and that people with such conditions may not absorb many of the nutrients needed to return them to good health. Also, many diseases cause the body to use nutrients at a faster rate, or to require higher amounts for proper healing. When nutrients are injected intravenously, the digestion is bypassed. Furthermore, the levels in the bloodstream are temporarily increased so that the nutrients are "coaxed" into the cells, and frequently into the mitochondria where they are active. This temporary boost frequently "kick-starts" the cells, so that energy is produced more efficiently in them.

Many chronic conditions respond to a series of Myers Cocktails. In my experience, they are useful in fibromyalgia, chronic fatigue syndrome, and chronic depression, where patients feel an energy boost lasting days or weeks. In the case of fibromyalgia, decreased pain can be observed. In other chronic conditions such as rheumatoid arthritis and ulcerative colitis, there is electron microscope evidence that the gut "leaks" nutrients, and the injections help get necessary nutrients into the cells. Chronic asthma and other lung disease, congestive heart failure, and chronic allergic problems can respond with more energy and less symptoms. Patients who get sick constantly with infections may find an increased immune response, with less susceptibility to in acute situations such as viral illnesses. The usual composition of the Myers Cocktail is:

1. B complex..1 cc

2. Vitamin C...1-10 cc or more, usually 222 mg/cc or 500 mg/cc

3. Magnesium...1-4 cc either 20% chloride or 50% sulfate

4. Dexpanthenol (B5)..1- 2cc

5. Calcium...1-4cc (sometimes not given in cardiac problems or in older patients)

Frequent additions are:

1. B12...1 cc

2. B6...1cc

3. Adrenal Cortical Extract (ACE).............................1-2 cc

4. Glyceron (an extract of licorice called glycerrhizin).... 1-2cc

5. Glutathione (an anti- oxidant)..............................1-2 cc

The latter three are not FDA approved and thus cannot be imported by physicians across state lines for the purpose of treating patients. The injections are diluted to 20 or 30 cc, more if there is increased vitamin C which tends to be thicker. A butterfly needle is then inserted into a vein, and the injection is given very slowly, at 1-2 cc per minute. Side effects are remarkably rare and almost always are limited to local irritation of the vein.

Allergy to the preservative in the nutrients must be tested for. The most common sensations are heat and flushing (a magnesium effect), and the taste of vitamins soon after the injection is begun. The injections are usually given 1-2 times per week, and beneficial effects are usually felt by the fourth shot.

Many patients with chronic conditions choose to continue the injections every 1-4 weeks or when they feel their energy slipping.

Why aren't more physicians using this therapy with wide applications and a strong record of safety?

First of all, most of them haven't heard of it. There are no studies of the Myers Cocktail, though Spectrum Medical Arts of Arlington, MA is planning to begin a study of the cocktail in fibromyalgia this fall. There are studies supporting the need for injectable magnesium and other nutrients in asthma, heart disease, and other chronic conditions. Another reason is the bias in medicine against nutritional treatments of illnesses, borne of the fact that pharmaceutical companies support much of the research in medical therapies, and no drug company will fund a study looking at the effects of simple vitamin shots. Also, there is a tendency to look for single ingredient therapies (for instance, vitamin C for the common cold) and the cocktail works better, in the opinion of its proponents, than using the nutrients individually.

Finally, old habits die hard in medicine, and the habit of reaching for a prescription pad for every illness will die harder than most. However, the need to look for safe, inexpensive therapies for chronic illnesses is becoming urgent under managed care insurance systems and it is possible that the Myers Cocktail will be re- discovered as a good example of this.

Environmental Factors in Autoimmune Disease

Environmental Health Perspectives: Questions Persist:

Environmental Factors in Autoimmune Disease ehp03.niehs.nih.gov

Environmental Health Perspectives (EHP) is a monthly journal of peer-reviewed research and news on the impact of the environment on human health. EHP is published by the National Institute of Environmental Health Sciences and its content is free online. Print issues are available by paid subscription

One reason why food and chemical allergy must be considered in evaluating health, and why you need healthy fat in your diet to protect you.

Device Eliminates Neuropathy Pain - How do I use the ReBuilder for neuropathy pain? Simply sit in your easy chair and turn on the ReBuilder www.rebuildermedical.com Drug free neuropathy treatment.

Benfotiamine or vitamin B1 (thiamine) since 1962 for diabetic neuropathy and to help with alcoholism treatment. Used in Europe since 1992, in the US since 2005. Found in roasted and crushed onions, shallots, garlic, leeks. Balances cellular sugar metabolism. Up to 1200 mg used safely. Many uses. Protects kidneys.

Diabetic Nutritional Supplement, Neuropathy Treatment, Benfotiamine, a derivative of vitamin b-1, has been used to alleviate diabetic complications, including neuropathy, retinopathy and nephropathy. Benfotiamine is an anti-AGE compound. Vitamin E will help this too according to Ray Peat, PhD, up to 1600-2000 IU daily.

SEANOL information - Brown algae extract containing polyphenols and phlorotannins which offers metabolic benefits of long duration and is highly bioavailable. Comes from research at the University of Iowa (go Hawkeyes!) in the 80s. It is considered a flavonoid (antioxidant) with 8 rings whereas most have 3 rings. They are also fat soluble and can cross the blood-brain barrier with a half-life of 12 hours.

Good for hypertension and vascular disease, helps break down clots, reduces fibrinogen levels, improves blood flow, act as an ACE inhibitor, reduces plaque and rejuvenates damaged lining in blood vessels, improves nitric oxide levels, inhibits LDL oxidation, anti-inflammatory, reduces neuropathy by 40% is a short time, helps prevent cognitive impairment, helps in allergic lung disease, helps with arthritis, helps fibromyalgia, inhibits aldose reductase to prevent damage to eyes-nerves etc in people with diabetes (helps reduce sugar alcohols or Sorbitol) helps reduce triclyderides, reduces fat in the pancreas to help insulin production, helps weight loss, AND, no side effects like Rx. CHI does have pharmaceutical grade Seanol products and many others as listed in Dr Jim's list. Profit from all sales supports our work.

Extract of Salacia oblonga lowers acute glycemia in patients with type 2 diabetes

American Journal of Clinical Nutrition, Vol. 86, No. 1, 124-130, July 2007. Jennifer A Williams, Yong S Choe, Michael J Noss, Carl J Baumgartner and Vikkie A Mustad. From the Ross Products Division of Abbott Laboratories, Columbus, OH; Radiant Research, Cincinnati, OH, and Radiant Research, Edina, MN.

This study evaluated the effect of an herbal extract of Salacia oblonga on postprandial glycemia and insulinemia in patients with type 2 diabetes after ingestion of a high-carbohydrate meal. Sixty-six patients with diabetes were studied in this randomized, double-blinded crossover study. In a fasted state, subjects consumed 1 of the following 3 meals: a standard liquid control meal, a control meal + 240 mg Salacia oblonga extract, and a control meal + 480 mg Salacia oblonga extract. Both doses of the Salacia extract significantly lowered the postprandial positive area under the glucose curve (14% for the 240 mg extract and 22% for the 480 mg extract) and the adjusted peak glucose response (19% for the lower dose and 27% for the higher dose of extract) to the control meal. In addition, both doses of the salacia extract significantly decreased the postprandial insulin response, lowering both the positive area under the insulin curve and the adjusted peak insulin response (14% and 9%, respectively, for the 240 mg extract; 19% and 12%, respectively, for the 480 mg extract) in comparison with the control meal.

My good friend and good doctor, Dr Jim Bowen, sends along some supplement information for people with diabetes (PWD)

Diabetes is probably helped by several extrinsic factors:

1. Androgen supplantation; which is well recognized as beneficial, and is badly needed, on a continuous basis.

2. Bentiamine (vit B1, active form bentofiamine and it helps protect your kidneys- GE) is a well recognized healer of neuropathy: Which is observed to help regenerate neuropathy damaged neurons:by eliminating excess levels of

potentially damaging glucose metabolites: (triosephposphates) Does this by increasing transketolase activity by about 400%. It has no known drug interactions.

3 ReBuilder: Which sends a non painful electrical stimulus which wakes up dormant neurons: Restores blood flow in those neurons;.

4. Chromium supplementation (chromium GTF or nicotinate - GE)

5. Bitter Melon Shown to reduce diabetic neuropathy within 5 hours.

6. Gymnema Sylvestre: Increases pancreatic production of insulin, by repairing pancreatic B cls, which produce insulin. And has no known side effects.

6. Niacinamide known since 1950s (vitamin B3 in the non-flush form also known as nicotinamide.) which prohibit immune attack on Beta Cells and increases the numbers of functional Beta Cells, and restores their activity.

7. Niacinamide: effective in preventing and treating diabetes: Stimulates the production of insulin restores beta cell and protects them from

immune attack. (dose is 25mg/ Kg) (also is good to reverse rheumatoid arthritis and help with fetal alcohol syndrome - GE)

8. Banaba (Corosilic acid the name given its active ingredient) ("Glucofit" is 18% corosilic acid.)

9. Salacia Oblongata in dose 1-5 Gms decreases both insulin and blood sugar levels.

10. Vanadyl Sulphate: (Which I personally found to toxic to my skin.) has been shown permanently eliminate diabetes in some.(In Europe this is used but the doses have to be in the toxic range so I do not usually suggest it -GE)

11. Resveratrol: Prevents many of the adverse effects of diabetes.(from grapeseed and grapeskin, grapes-GE)

12. Seanol: Shown effective: Treating neuropathy (I take 11 and 12 every day) ((An algae, Ecklonina cava. I'll post more on this-GE))

MAY 2011

This advice comes from a Diabetes newsletter, amazing! These are suggested candy bars for people with diabetes. The Happiness Cure for Diabetes

Tip of the Week - The Candy Bar of Choice for Diabetes

Alongside the checkout aisle, a multitude of candy bars tempt you with the sweet taste of childhood memories. You've recently checked your blood sugar and know that you have a few calories to splurge on a snack. But which bar is best? They all contain lots of sugar and calories. Here, we decode three of the most popular bars so you can evaluate your indulgence:

• Snickers (30 g sugar, 280 calories, 4 g protein) scores as the best of the worst. Even though it's slightly higher in calories than other bars, it contains the lowest amount of sugar. Snickers also packs in nuts, a source of fiber and healthy monounsaturated fat. And compared to the non-nutty bars, Snickers will slightly curb the blood-sugar spike you'll experience after munching one.

• Milky Way (35 g sugar, 260 calories, 2 g protein) consists mostly of marshmallowy fluff and caramel, so it's digested rapidly—which is what causes those rollercoaster blood-sugar spikes and dips. On the plus side, though, Milky Way offers the most calcium of the three at 6 percent of Recommended Daily Value.

• 3 Musketeers (40 g sugar, 260 calories, 2 g protein) commercials show the bars floating away because they're so light. But it's high sugar content and negligible amount of fiber—only 1 g—makes it the worst choice of the three.

CHI started reporting on EMF and cancer in the late 90s. This information has been known since the 1940s. People need to wake up to the fact that there is a real risk of cancer from cell phones. Also implicated in diabetes, asthma, breast cancer and more.

Many people with diabetes (PWD) are told they must take statin drugs. For the most part this is not a beneficial pharmaceutical and it has high risk for PWD. Statin drugs - In January of 2008 results from a study sponsored by Merck and Schering-Plough that found that after several years on two types of cholesterol-lowering medications, patients reduced their cholesterol level, but they reaped no significant health benefit at all unless they already had heart disease. (Note: Merck delayed releasing the results for two years, and only when finally pressed to do so.) Worldwide this ineffective class of drugs accounts for revenues exceeding $26 billion in 2008 alone. And they are hardly without risk, having been associated with a 50% increased risk of cancer of all kinds, structural damage to muscles, and cataract and kidney risk. (JB)

The Importance of Fiber

Health Benefits of Psyllium Seed Husk www.leaflady.org

7 grams of fiber daily in the form of psyllium can help lower cholesterol without drugs which have very serious risk of side effects for people with diabetes. If you use psyllium use the husk and not processed products like Metamucil. Metamucil uses aspartame, artificial colors, and other additives, and it is owned by a Big PhRMA firm. A tablespoon of organic psyllium in water, followed by a glass of filtered water is a food addition to your regular daily supplement regimen. This plain psyllium husk powder is much healthier than processed products and will cost much less. Capsules are also available or you can make your own capsules easily. For better nutrient benefit the Ayurvedic herbal combination Triphala is a good choice. There is information about Triphala linked to my psyllium web page.

Cinnamon

Before insulin, botanical medicines were used to treat diabetes. They are remarkably safe and effective. However, because many botanical medicines function similarly to insulin, people taking oral diabetes medications or insulin should use caution to avoid hypoglycemia. Botanical medicines should be integrated into a regimen of adequate exercise, healthy eating, nutritional supplements, and medical support. From LEF.

Prevent Neuropathy with Vitamin E and BioSupplemente

Consumer Reports: Expert product reviews and product Ratings from our test labs www.consumerreports.org

On this site look for Nerve damage in diabetes

Over time, high levels of glucose (sugar) in your blood can stop your nerves from sending signals from your limbs (especially your legs and feet) to your brain. Other nerves, called autonomic nerves, also can get damaged. Autonomic nerves control many functions in your body, such as your heartbeat, digestion and blood pressure.

About half of people who have had diabetes for a long time get some kind of nerve damage. 1 This nerve damage is called diabetic neuropathy. http://www.consumerreports.org/health/conditions-andtreatments/

diabetes-type-2/what-will-happen/nerve-damage-in-diabetes.htm

Broccoli sprouts show benefits for people with diabetes Broccoli sprouts show benefits for diabetics: RCT

www.nutraingredients.com Powdered broccoli sprouts may boost antioxidant defenses in people with diabetes, suggest findings from a randomized clinical trial from Iran.

The Soft Science of Dietary Fat, and YES, you do need it. http://www.gunnarlindgren.com/nutritionx.pdf

www.gunnarlindgren.com Important to know about fat because low fat and no fat diets can kill you.

The Importance of CO Q 10, especially if using toxic statin drugs
Statins destroy COQ10 and this is important for your heart.

Cooked tomatoes 'as good as statins' for battling cholesterol. Great
news for people with Diabetes. www.dailymail.co.uk

Scientists said that cooked tomatoes can have the same benefits as
statins for patients battling against high cholesterol levels or high blood
pressure.

Statin drugs are very dangerous and can lead to kidney failure. Cooked
tomatoes also benefit prostate health.

GMO Toxins in Blood of Unborn Babies

GM food toxins found in the blood of 93% of unborn babies
www.dailymail.co.uk

A landmark study found 93 per cent of blood samples taken from
pregnant women and 80 per cent from umbilical cords tested positive
for traces of the chemicals.

Toxins implanted into GM food crops to kill crop pests are reaching
the bloodstreams of women & unborn babies, research reveals. The
study was by independent doctors at the Dept of Obstetrics &
Gynaecology at the University of Sherbrooke Hospital Centre in
Quebec, Canada. The landmark study found 93% of blood samples
taken from pregnant women & 80% from umbilical cords tested
positive for traces of the chemicals. Millions of acres in North & South
America are planted with GM corn containing the toxins, which is fed
in vast quantities to farm livestock around the world - including UK.

There is speculation it could lead to allergies, miscarriage, abnormalities
& cancer. The industry always argued that if these toxins were eaten by
animals or humans they would be destroyed in the gut. Food safety
authorities in UK & Europe accepted these assurances.

But the latest study appears to disprove this & has triggered calls for a ban on imports & a total overhaul of the safety regime for GM. Most of the research used to demonstrate GM safety has been funded by the industry itself. It now appears the proteins can survive the digestive system & pass into the bloodstream. The toxins in the blood were Bt toxins implanted using GM techniques into corn & some other crops. Traces were found in 69% of the non-pregnant group. They are thought to be getting into the body as a result of eating meat, milk & eggs from farm livestock fed GM corn.

Published in "Reproductive Toxicology." They said the Bt toxin was "clearly detectable & appears to cross the placenta to the foetus."

'GM Freeze' group called for safeguard clauses in the regulations to be used to prevent any further GMBt crops being cultivated or imported for animal feed or food until the health implications are fully evaluated. RoundUp has some Agent Orange ingredients and this is liked to diabetes.

From and orthomolecular pioneer -

Eating a High Protein Breakfast for Better Health Eat high-protein breakfast, eat less later Published: May 20, 2011 at 1:28 AM

COLUMBIA, Mo., May 20 (UPI) -- People who eat a healthy breakfast - especially one high in protein - are more full and are less hungry throughout the day, U.S. researchers found.

Heather Leidy, an assistant professor at the University of Missouri, says people may have an easier time preventing weight gain by eating a healthy, protein-rich breakfast such as waffles made with protein powder.

"Everyone knows that eating breakfast is important, but many people still don't make it a priority," Leidy says in a statement. "This research provides additional evidence that breakfast is a valuable strategy to control appetite and regulate food intake."

For three weeks, teens in the study either skipped breakfast or consumed 500-calorie breakfast meals containing cereal and milk, which contained normal quantities of protein, or higher protein meals such as the protein-added Belgium waffles, syrup and yogurt.

At the end of each week, the volunteers completed appetite and satiety questionnaires and before lunch, the volunteers completed a brain scan, using functional magnetic resonance imaging to identify brain activation responses, Leidy says.

The study, published in the journal Obesity, finds both breakfast meals led to increased fullness and reductions in hunger throughout morning The fMRI showed brain activation in regions controlling food motivation and reward was reduced prior to lunch.

Read more: http://www.upi.com/Health_News/2011/05/20/Eat-high-protein-breakfast-eat-lesslater/

UPI-48111305869321/print/#ixzz1MuxVJyRA

The Importance of Sleep and Blood Sugar Balance Getting adequate sleep appears to help insulin functioning and blood sugar control | Dr Briffa's Blog www.drbriffa.com

There was an interesting, I think, study published this week in which the association between sleep habits and certain metabolic processes were assessed.

Dr Briffa is one of the few doctors with an open mind and belief in natural approaches to health.

Food for the Health of Your Cells

bioSUPPLEMENTE at leaflady.org

Optimizes the body's use of energy - Reduces the risk of developing diabetes and heart disease Blood glucose - DKSH global www.dksh.com The remarkable range of health benefits of beta glucan is now well established. Central to many of these benefits is the ability of beta glucan to improve blood glucose control. Good control maintains healthy blood glucose levels and provides two key advantages:

Strawberries Promote Weight Loss Slimming Strawberries For Weight Loss www.huffingtonpost.com Red, ripe and delicious, strawberries are a little fruit that work overtime for your health. Peak strawberry season is just around the corner, so now is the perfect time to add strawberries to your menu for summer weight loss.

The important concern is to be sure to get organic berries because of the toxic chemicals used on standard berry crops. All berries are health promoting and contain high levels of anthocyanidins. The ellagic acid and anthocyanins found in strawberries aid weight loss in at least three ways:

Chronic inflammation blocks the hormones involved in keeping you lean. Anti-inflammatory foods like strawberries help restore normal function to weight-reducing hormones.

Anthocyanins actually increase the body's production of a hormone called adiponectin, which stimulates your metabolism and suppresses your appetite.

Both ellagic acid and anthocyanins slow the rate of digestion of starchy foods, controlling the rise in blood sugar that follows a starchy meal. This effect is used to control blood sugar in people with adult onset (Type 2) diabetes.

3 Very Healthy Foods Among the healthiest foods on the planet, these are high in the fiber and nutrients that are perfect for healthy blood sugar and metabolism. Not to mention, they're hearty and delicious. Here's how to cook with them.

Barley: Use it as an alternative for pasta or rice, or sauté it with veggies for a side dish. Chill it and make a barley salad with herbs, dressing, and a sprinkling of Parmesan cheese. Barley water is a survival food. Barley has plenty of health promoting B vitamins and it has beta glucan which boosts immunity. It is in our BioSupplemente.

Bran: Use it to replace half the flour in muffin recipes. Mix it into meat loaf or sprinkle bran flakes on casseroles. Oat bran is a best choice. Wheat bran can deplete iron.

Bulgur: (also called kasha) Make bulgur pilaf as a side dish or use the grain cold to make a salad such as tabbouleh. Cook hot bulgur cereal in salted water as you would oatmeal.

How walking can help you prevent diabetes More information is a thttp://www.rodale.com/howprevent-diabetes?page=0%2C0

Do something for your best health - Make a pact to be as healthy as possible, to reduce the money you spend on medical and long-term care bills. Get daily exercise, walk together after dinner. Make healthy food, band together to grow your own food in a vegetable garden. Use herbs and supplements. Many of these do better than drugs, just ask.

Pet Health - Prevent Diabetes for them too. Fat Cats, Dogs Developing Diabetes, Report Finds

By Maryann Mott, HealthDay Reporter

FRIDAY, May 13 (HealthDay News) -- Like all good pet owners, Christine Wong didn't hesitate to go to a veterinary clinic near her home in Austin, Texas, when her cat, Kiki, wasn't feeling well.

"She just wasn't acting like herself," recalled Wong.

After running a blood and urine test, the doctor discovered the Persian-mix feline has diabetes.

Diabetes is on the rise as America's cats and dogs grow fatter, according to a new report by Banfield Pet Hospital, a national chain of pet hospitals headquartered in Portland, Ore. Since 2006, diabetes jumped 32 percent in dogs and 16 percent in cats, says the report, which analyzed trends in common and preventable illnesses from the past five years.

Just as in people, diabetes is often linked to obesity and may require lifelong monitoring and treatment.

"The most important thing we can do for a cat with diabetes is getting it on a weight loss program," said Dr. Denise Elliott, a veterinarian with Banfield.

"We know that if we can get the weight off in conjunction with insulin injections, in many cases we can resolve the cat's diabetes," she added.

Fat cats are six times more likely to develop diabetes than their thinner feline cousins, Elliott said.

For the report, researchers crunched data from the records of 2.5 million dogs and cats cared for last year in its 770 hospitals nationwide.

Symptoms of diabetes in both dogs and cats may include excessive urination, increased thirst and weight loss, despite a hearty appetite. If not detected and treated early, dogs in advanced stages of the disease might develop cataracts and cats may experience hind-limb weakness, Elliott said.

There are two types of diabetes mellitus. Dogs often get type 1 (insulin-dependent), which is similar to the form seen in children, in which the pancreas produces little or no insulin, a hormone that helps cells turn sugar into energy. Breeds prone to the condition are bichon frise, cairn terrier, dachshund, keeshond, miniature poodle and puli.

Cats are commonly affected by type 2 diabetes, or non-insulin dependent, in which the pancreas produces insulin but the body does not respond normally to it. At-risk breeds include Maine coon, Russian blue and Siamese.

For dogs with diabetes, it's usually a lifelong battle. Along with a special diet, they typically need insulin injections twice a day, veterinarians say. Once clinical signs resolve, blood glucose concentrations are monitored every three to four months to determine if changes to the treatment plan are necessary.

But the outlook for dogs is good. "Typically dogs that are treated properly for diabetes go on to live a long, full life," said Dr. Charles Wiedmeyer, assistant professor of veterinary clinical pathology at the University of Missouri in Columbia.

Wiedmeyer and colleague Dr. Amy DeClue, assistant professor of veterinary internal medicine, recently adapted a device used to monitor glucose in humans to help dogs with diabetes that don't respond well to conventional treatment. Continuous glucose monitors (CGM) are flexible devices inserted an inch or so into the skin to provide detailed information on sugar levels.

Using a CGM, a dog's blood sugar levels can be monitored at home in everyday situations rather than in a cage at the animal hospital, they say. Normally, veterinarians create an insulin regimen by taking blood from the animal in the clinic every two hours over the course of a single day. But test results are often inaccurate, he said, because of stress felt by pets from being in an unfamiliar environment.

Adapting to the needs of a diabetic pet isn't easy. When Kiki, Wong's cat, was diagnosed three years ago with diabetes, the toughest part was getting used to giving the insulin shots, Wong said.

Now it's a breeze, she noted. Kiki receives insulin injections every 12 hours -- before Wong leaves for work and when she returns home -- plus occasional check-ups and a modified diet.

It costs Wong about $65 a month to manage her pet's disease. But she doesn't mind the added cost or extra time spent in caring for Kiki.

"In the end, she and I are definitely closer for all of it," said Wong. "She lives well and seems healthy and happy these days, far from the end. And this makes it all worth it."

More information - You can find out more about managing diabetes in your pet at the Washington State University College of Veterinary Medicine.

Remember your pets need a healthy diet too and most pet foods are too high in carbs, contain toxic ingredients. Don't overlook the vaccines issue in your pet's health too as they may cause diabetes as they do for humans.

See the Pet Health pages at leaflady.org

Diabetes drug Actos linked to higher risk of bladder cancer. More signs diabetes drug linked to bladder cancer news.yahoo.com

A review of official reports of bad drug reactions is revealing more signs that people taking the diabetes drug Actos are at higher risk of developing bladder cancer.

Vitamin C in high doses is good for issues relating to bladder cancer. Adults should be at a minimum of 3-4000 mg daily for basic intake.

Diabetes Diet v. Paleolithic Diet. Paleo diet wins hands down for PWD. Paleolithic diet much better for diabetics than conventional 'diabetes diet' | Dr Briffa's Blog – A. www.drbriffa.com

Over the weekend I spent some time looking at the evidence in the area of 'primal' or 'Paleolithic' eating. I was aware, I think, of much of the Paleo diet – Dr Phil Bate, orthomolecular pioneer, Paleo .com

How Garlic Oil May Help People with Diabetes - The study, published in the Journal of Agricultural and Food Chemistry, suggests that cardiac abnormalities induced by diabetes can be reversed in as little sixteen days of garlic oil supplementation. The great thing is that this is easy to make and it is super easy to grow your own organic garlic. Just pack a glass jar full with peeled and cracked garlic cloves and fill jar with high quality olive oil or sesame seed oil, cap and shake well. Set in the cupboard and shake daily, do this for 7-14 days, strain and there you have it. Eat the garlic or use for cooking.

April 2011

Strawberries help lower blood sugar

Hazards from Splenda: not for use by people with diabetes.

Consider the cost of nutrition-related disease. $4 trillion that Republicans want cut is about the same as the projected costs of diabetes over that same period. See low fruit and vegetable intake, also recall that in the 70s and 80s the push was on to use more margarine, local foods, and cut real fat from your diet. Plus Big AG is more in control of USDA so dietitians (RD) are spoon fed this pablum rather than sound nutritional information.

Diet Can Reverse Kidney Damage. Diet 'can reverse kidney failure' www.bbc.co.uk

A diet high in fat and low in carbohydrate can repair damaged kidneys in diabetic mice, according to US scientists.

Vitamin B1 in adequate amounts helps this too. Many get an Rx for anti-hypertensives to protect kidneys but they too have side effects risks.

Nutrient supplementation helps symptoms of diabetic neuropathy Vitamin E, Sesame Seed oil. This is from a like minded medical professional in the UK. All of the supplements listed can help but vitamin E(mixed tocopherols) are a good place to start.

http://www.drbriffa.com/category/diabetesmetabolic-syndrome/

Pecans are high in tocopherols (related to vitamin E) and seem to lower HDL.

Pecans may lower bad cholesterol Published: April 21, 2011LOMA LINDA, Calif., April 21 (UPI) -- A handful of pecans each day may boost antioxidant levels in the body and help protect the heart, California researchers suggest.

Dr. Ella Haddad, associate professor at the School of Public Health at Loma Linda University in California, says pecans contain different forms of the antioxidant vitamin E, known as tocopherols, and the nuts are especially rich in one form of vitamin E called gamma-tocopherols.

This type of antioxidant has been shown to double in the human body after eating pecans and it may lead to a decrease in bad cholesterol, Haddad says.

The study, published in The Journal of Nutrition, finds testing conducted after participants had eaten pecans showed gamma-tocopherols doubled and oxidation of low-density lipoprotein, LDL or 'bad cholesterol', decreased by one-third.

"This study confirms previous research which shows pecans are a healthy food," Haddad says in a statement. "Our study indicates that antioxidants in pecans are absorbed in the body and provide a protective effect against the development of various diseases such as cancer and heart disease."

Learning that a doctor at a Pullman WA health clinic is still ignorant of the facts about vitamin E is not surprising but certainly absurd when the real science shows those studies to have been poorly constructed and they utilized synthetic vitamin E in extremely low doses. Vitamin E does not cause cancer and it will prevent and reverse heart disease, plus much more. You must use natural and mixed forms, not synthetic.

Why Your Thyroid Should Work Properly

Arsenic in water linked to Diabetes risk Could Arsenic Exposure From Drinking Water Cause Type 2 diabetes?

Arsenic Exposure and Prevalence of Type 2 Diabetes in US Adults.

CONTEXT: High chronic exposure to inorganic arsenic in drinking water has been related to diabetes development, but the effect of exposure to low to moderate levels of inorganic arsenic on diabetes risk is unknown. In contrast, arsenobetaine, an organic arsenic compound derived from seafood intake, is considered nontoxic.

OBJECTIVE: To investigate the association of arsenic exposure, as measured in urine, with the prevalence of type 2 diabetes in a representative sample of US adults.

DESIGN, SETTING, AND PARTICIPANTS: Cross-sectional study in 788 adults aged 20 years or older who participated in the 2003-2004 National Health and Nutrition Examination Survey (NHANES) and had urine arsenic determinations.

MAIN OUTCOME MEASURE: Prevalence of type 2 diabetes across intake of arsenic.

RESULTS: The median urine levels of total arsenic, dimethylarsinate, and arsenobetaine were 7.1, 3.0, and 0.9 mug/L, respectively. The prevalence of type 2 diabetes was 7.7%. After adjustment for diabetes risk factors and markers of seafood intake, participants with type 2 diabetes had a 26% higher level of total arsenic (95% confidence interval [CI], 2.0%-56.0%) and a nonsignificant 10% higher level of dimethylarsinate (95% CI, -8.0% to 33.0%) than participants without type 2 diabetes, and levels of arsenobetaine were similar to those of participants without type 2 diabetes. After similar adjustment, the odds ratios for type 2 diabetes comparing participants at the 80th vs the 20th percentiles were 3.58 for the level of total arsenic (95% CI, 1.18-10.83), 1.57 for dimethylarsinate (95% CI, 0.89-2.76), and 0.69 for arsenobetaine (95% CI, 0.33-1.48).

CONCLUSIONS: After adjustment for biomarkers of seafood intake, total urine arsenic was associated with increased prevalence of type 2 diabetes. This finding supports the hypothesis that low levels of exposure to inorganic arsenic in drinking water, a widespread exposure worldwide, may play a role in diabetes prevalence. Prospective studies in populations exposed to a range of inorganic arsenic levels are needed to establish whether this association is causal.

Sources / Credits: Department of Environmental Health Sciences, Johns Hopkins Bloomberg School of Public Health, 615 N Wolfe St, Room W7033B, Baltimore, MD 21205, USA. anavas@jhsph.edu and www.pubmed.gov, www.ncbi.nlm.nih.gov

I generally recommend to people with diabetes to use digestive enzymes and probiotics. Here is some support from new research.

Aspartame and Diabetes Aspartame can precipitate diabetes, simulates and aggravates diabetic retinopathy and neuropathy, destroys the optic nerve, interacts with insulin and causes diabetics to go into convulsions. The free methyl alcohol causes diabetics to lose limbs. You must get her off of it. It may be difficult because its so addicting. The methyl alcohol is classified as a narcotic, causes chronic methanol poisoning and this affects the dopamine system of the brain causing the addiction. I just sent you the Aspartame Resource Guide and it contained Dr. H. J. Roberts medical text, Aspartame Disease: An Ignored Epidemic. Dr. Roberts, the world expert on aspartame, is a diabetic specialist and besides the information above has a whole chapter on diabetes. You need to get this medical text, and if your mother won't get off of it you need to show it to her physician so he will understand and help her somehow. Also, read this letter from Dr. Bowen on the subject: http://www.wnho.net/letter_to_senator_goyp_concerning_aspartame. htm

DMG (Di-METHYL-glycine) DMG is anti cancer in high doses, supplies O2 which cancer cells do not like 1500-2500mg daily. It helps protect even with chemo and radiation, other. It is also helpful for diabetes.

Oxygen (O2) is the key and it is a methyl donor.

Say NO to Aspartame: The 'Hidden' Danger Say NO to Aspartame: The 'Hidden' Danger - Arab News arabnews.com

Round Up and other chemicals are linked to diabetes too - New pathogen found in Roundup Ready crops casually linked to miscarriages and spontaneous abortions in farm animals. "Unknown Organism"

Linked to Roundup Ready Crops uk.ibtimes.com

Carbohydrate sweeteners must be labelled for gastric distress in the EU - The NDA found sugar replacers can decrease tooth demineralisation if four foods-drinks are consumed daily but not below 5.7. Xylitol, sorbitol, mannitol, maltitol, lactitol, isomalt, erythritol, D-tagatose, isomaltulose, sucralose and polydextrose containing products must include "excessive consumption may produce laxative effects" disclaimer. EFSA sweetens industry with positive sugar replacement health claim opinions www.nutraingredients.com

Intense and bulk sweetener suppliers are basking in the glow of positive sugar replacement health claim opinions issued by the European Food Safety Authority (EFSA) last week.

2008, Natural Health News -http://bit.ly/cdGUTI

Only 6% of PWD lose their vision. Blindness is largely preventableby working together diligently with your health provider. Prevention relies upon the proper use of medications, daily blood sugar testing, correct lifestyle habits, diet and supplements. Certain nutrients help those with diabetic retinopathy and may help to preserve vision. Diabetic Retinopathy (macular edema or proliferative macular degeneration): cause, prevention, treat www.naturaleyecare.com Diabetic retinopathy is a potentially blinding complication of diabetes that damages the eye's retina. It affects half of all Americans diagnosed with diabetes.

Tangerines - Good for Health Citrus peel extract shows benefits for diabetes http://www.nutraingredients.com/Research/Citrus-peel-extract-shows-benefits-for-diabetes A flavonoid found in tangerines may not only prevents obesity, but may protect against type-2 diabetes, and atherosclerosis, suggests new research.

People with Diabetes (PWD) are at higher risk for mineral deficiencies compared to the general public.

When blood sugar is elevated they pass large amounts of urine, which contains valuable minerals and nutrients.

Some diabetes medication causes nutrient depletion too. Metformin depletes vitamin B12.

Supplements for PWD - daily intake of the following nutrients chromium 1000 to 2000 mg., Niacin 1.5 to 2.5 mg , Niacinamide 50 to 100 mg , Biotin 8 to 16 mg., Alpha-lipoic- acid 300 mg., Co-Enzyme Q 10-60 mg., Vitamin K 5 to 10 mg., Vitamin D -2000 I.U. daily, Vitamin E (as mixed tocopherols) 400 IU, Vitamin C 2000-3000 mg., Magnesium 300-400 mg., Vanadium 1-2 mg., Zinc 30 mg. Copper 2 mg., Manganese 5-10 mg., omega 3. I often encourage 10K of vit C daily and also up to 1600IU vit E, probitotics and others depending on if you use Metformin or insulin, other drugs. Selenium in the correct form.

Alcohol causes severe nutrient depletion. This is one reason why alcoholics are at greater risk of developing cancers and diabetes, et al.

Health Impact Study III Shows Supplements Help Better Manage Diabetes

Successfully controlling diabetes is complicated, and a new study indicates that diabetics who take dietary supplements, while following other healthy behaviors, feel healthier and look after themselves better. Vitamin E (natural, non soy) can prevent and reverse peripheral neuropathy when using the right dose.

Help from Bitter Melon to Balance Blood Sugar

Of all of the botanical powerhouses available to you in your efforts to support healthy blood sugar, Momordica charantis—also known as "bitter melon"—is among the most revered. Supported by centuries of traditional use and decades of scientific research, bitter melon is a must-have if you want to maintain healthy glucose levels.

But what if you want to enhance memory, maintain healthy motor skills and support your brain's neurons for peak functioning long-term? According to one recent study, bitter melon may still be among your best natural solutions.

As part of this new study, researchers supplemented a group of mice with Momordica juice at dosages ranging between 200 and 800 mg per kilogram of body weight. The carotid arteries of the mice were then exposed to suboptimal blood flow for ten minutes, during which the brain didn't receive sufficient oxygen-rich blood. The researchers then restored optimal blood flow through the carotid arteries of the mice for 24 hours.

Since optimal blood flow restoration is known to increase the generation of free radicals in previously oxygen-deprived tissues, scientists evaluated the mice for blood levels of thiobarbituric acid (TBA) reactive substances, a marker of oxidative stress. In addition to free radical generation, researchers looked for any effects on the neurological performance of the mice, including motor skill and shortterm memory function.

This experiment's results revealed an incredibly promising trend: The mice previously supplemented with Momordica juice fared significantly better with respect to both oxidative stress levels and cognitive performance than mice that had not received Momordica juice. What's more, these effects appeared to be dose-dependent—indicating that higher intake of bitter melon juice delivers proportionately higher protection against free radicals and supports neurological health.1

Finally, researchers also observed Momordica juice's positive influence on blood glucose levels—leading to their conclusion that bitter melon has benefits to the brain health of mice that have unbalanced blood sugar metabolism.

If this recent animal study is any indication of the benefits of this botanical in humans, a daily dose of bitter melon could turn out to help support both healthy blood sugar levels and your brain, too. You can find Momordica charantia in some of the high quality supplements we offer.

Reference:

1. Malik ZA, Singh M, Sharma PL. Neuroprotective effect of Momordica charantia in global cerebral ischemia and reperfusion induced neuronal damage in diabetic mice. Ethnopharmacol. 2010 Nov 5.

Published Online Ahead of Print.

Inflammation, Diabetes, Smoking, Blood Sugar, and A1C - Smoking raises all these parameters.

Important diabetes and inflammation issue, food allergy also; 38% of Native people have this reaction.

Genetic clues to major cause of kidney disease worldwide www.sciencedaily.com For the first time, researchers have found five regions in the human genome that increase susceptibility to immunoglobulin A (IgA) nephropathy, a major cause of kidney failure worldwide – systematically identifying those that point to a tendency for IgA nephropathy, or a protection against it.

More on Liver Health

ORLANDO, Fla., April 6 (UPI) -- Metabolic syndrome, conditions which increase heart disease and diabetes risk, may also increase liver cancer risk, U.S. researchers suggest.

Katherine McGlynn, a senior investigator at the National Cancer Institute, said approximately one-third of the U.S. population has metabolic syndrome -- at least three of five conditions: raised blood pressure, elevated waist circumference, low high-density lipoprotein or "good" cholesterol, raised triglyceride levels and raised fasting plasma glucose levels.

The study found people with metabolic syndrome may be at increased risk of developing hepatocellular carcinoma and intrahepatic cholangiocarcinoma -- two types of liver cancer.

"The prognosis for liver cancer is only marginally better than the prognosis for pancreatic cancer, with a five-year survival of approximately 10 percent," McGlynn says in a statement. "Prognosis is more favorable, however, when liver cancers are diagnosed at early stages when they are small and localized to the liver."

The researchers conducted statistical analyses involving 3,649 cases of hepatocellular carcinoma and 743 cases of intrahepatic cholangiocarcinoma and 195,953 cancer-free controls that showed people with liver cancer were significantly more likely than cancer-free people to have a prior history of metabolic syndrome.

McGlynn says 37.1 percent of patients with hepatocellular carcinoma had pre-existing metabolic syndrome, as did 29.7 percent of patients with intraheptic carcinoma, vs. 17.1 percent of the cancer free adults had metabolic syndrome.

The findings were presented at the American Association for Cancer Research's 102nd annual meeting in Orlando, Fla.

Read more: http://www.upi.com/Health_News/2011/04/06/Liver-cancer-linked-to-metabolicsyndrome/

UPI-22041302063559/#ixzz1Il9F4cbz

One reason to use LIV 52 or Milk Thistle should you be a person with diabetes.

Native American health data and diabetes data sorely lacking

Measure of America: American Human Development Project www.measureofamerica.org The Measure of America is the first-ever human development report for a wealthy, developed nation. It introduces the American Human Development Index, which provides a single measure of well-being for all Americans, disaggregated by state and congressional district, as well as by gender, race, and Best Exercise plan for people with Diabetes. Found this site with some good resources. Diabetes weight loss workout www.jarretmorrow.com What's the best workout or training program for those with type 2 diabetes who're looking to improve their blood sugar control and lose weight and belly fat?

I discovered years ago while researching my initial natural program for diabetes that especially for Plains tribes, diabetes was a survival mechanism. Now that concept related to starvation levels is resurfacing but related to poor quality food and Rx.

How the Biology of Starvation Contributes to Disease

What often happens in poverty-stricken families is a hunger-bingeing cycle that follows the economic conditions in the household. When resources come in, people buy cheap, abundant calories in the form of junk and processed foods that fill them up and stave off hunger. This leads to rapid fat storage —a common biological effect after a period of lower calorie intake or hunger. This is simply how human metabolism works.

When calories are scarce metabolism slows down and muscle is lost. As a result the blood sugar imbalances that drive the process of insulin resistance and lead to pre-diabetes and diabetes [3] worsens, and soon people are caught in a recurrent pattern of bingeing on nutrient-poor calories once resources are again available.

Certainly people can learn to eat better for less [6] as I pointed out in my recent blog on the topic, and doing so is an essential part of what needs to happen to break out of this cycle of poverty and disease as I will discuss more below. That said, breaking the hunger-binge cycle is easier said than done. Bingeing after food scarcity and the increased fat accumulation and insulin resistance that come along with it are hard-wired biological mechanisms to prevent us from starvation. Once you have diabetes, engaging in this cycle makes blood sugar control that much more difficult and leads to the swings of high and low sugar that drive health problems and their related costs.

Diabetics without access to adequate food have fives times as many doctor visits as diabetics who have enough to eat on a regular basis. The burden this creates in families already struggling to stay afloat is unspeakable. It's like they are caught in a Grecian hell—pushing the boulder of economic burden up a hill they will never see the top of, reaching for fruit that grows ever further from their reach.

We need to rethink how and what we feed our nation or the epidemics of disease and obesity will consume us. In Haiti, one in two people worry about where their next meal will come from. In America it is one in 10. In order to shift this we need a bold new vision and initiatives that can change our food culture and food availability.

http://drhyman.com/not-having-enough-food-causes-obesity-and-diabetes-2280/print/

Obesity in America: Are Factory Farms, Big Pharma and Big Food to Blame?

http://www.huffingtonpost.com/dr-mark-hyman/the-toxic-triad-how-big-f_b_772729.html?view=print

GMO Foods and drugs certainly contribute to disease
http://www.responsibletechnology.org/gmodangers/health-risks

More on protecting your liver

Learn to read labels, fructose in many forms is in almost everything. It also by-passes digestion so increases glucose levels quickly.

March 2011

NCAA sports new requirement for supplement and banned substance education. You can find help at Creating Health Institute and our new services from Health Forensics.

People with diabetes are 70% more likely to die from liver disease Liver failure is a great risk for people with diabetes and for those without the condition, 70% less likely to have problems according to new research.- I have more information on how to keep your liver healthy which in turn helps you have better control and lower blood sugar levels as well as better endocrine health overall.

This BBC article from today is helpful - It is already known that diabetes can increase the risk of some types of liver disease, with poor blood sugar control boosting the risk.

This can lead to scarring of the liver - also known as cirrhosis - and cancer.

In the study, Edinburgh researchers analysed the records of people aged 35 to 84 over a six-year period to 2007.

They compared 1,267 diabetes sufferers to 10,100 people without the condition, who all died of liver disease.

The results showed about one in four (24%) people with diabetes died of liver cancer, compared to one in ten (9%) of non-diabetics.

However, more people without diabetes died from alcoholic liver disease (63%) compared to those with diabetes (38%).

Diabetic patients are advised not to drink too much alcohol because of its potential impact on blood sugar levels and the risk of weight gain.

Dr Sarah Wild, of Edinburgh University, said: "Non-alcoholic fatty liver disease has become much more common recently, particularly among people with diabetes.

"The major risk factor for it is being overweight, which is also an important risk factor for Type 2 diabetes.

"Non-alcoholic fatty liver disease increases the risk of cirrhosis which in turn increases the risk of liver cancer.

"A healthy lifestyle can reduce the risk and prevention is particularly important because the options for treatment are limited."

The research is being presented at the Diabetes UK Annual Professional Conference, which ends on Friday.

Diabetes UK director of research, Dr Iain Frame, said: "Previous studies have found a link between diabetes and liver disease and this research adds to that knowledge.

"We now need further investigation into how diabetes affects the liver to find new methods of preventing this complication."

BBC © MMXI The BBC is not responsible for the content of Some of the diabetes drugs and insulins (GMO type) contribute to the development of fatty liver.

Nutritional deficiencies also play a role.

This could be a great resource Food Allergy Buddy archive.supermarketguru.com

More than 11 million Americans suffer from food allergies and predictions are that the incidence of food allergies is on the increase! One of the most awkward and embarrassing aspects of having food allergies is going to a restaurant and communicating which ingredients are problematic. Then the food...

Health professionals and the public should be aware of the great importance of Mg for insulin sensitivity and therefore, as a result, for the prevention of metabolic syndrome and type 2 diabetes. As a consequence, in obese subjects and in subjects with increased risk for metabolic syndrome and diabetes the Mg status should be optimized with supplementation. Magnesium (Mg) is important for anyone with diabetes.

People on a high-dose regimen of the cholesterol drug Lipitor may have a slightly increased risk of developing type 2 diabetes Predictors of New-Onset Diabetes in Patients Treated With Atorvastatin:

Results From 3 Large Randomized Trials content.onlinejacc.org

* Division of Cardiology, San Francisco General Hospital, and the University of California at San Francisco, San Francisco, California Pfizer, Inc., New York, New York Academic Medical Center, University of Amsterdam, Amsterdam, the Netherlands Department of Public Health, University of Dundee, Dund

Aspartame is Harmful to the Health of People with Diabetes
From Aspartame Disease: An Ignored Epidemic by H. J. Roberts, M.D.:

The Methyl Alcohol Syndrome:

"Eye damage (retinopathy)

"Methanol causes blindness, largely due to the toxic effects of formaldehyde and formic acid on the retina. Indeed, suspicion of "wood alcohol poisoning" was raised by ophthalmologist in several patients with aspartame disease.

"Formate, a metabolite of formaldehyde, probably induces retinal damage through energy depletion because it inhibit adenosine triphosphate (ATP).

"Edema of the optic disc (Hayreh 1977) and retinal ganglion cell degeneration (Baumbach 197) occur in monkeys poisoned with methanol.

Involvement of the peripheral nerves (neuropathy) "The symptoms include numbness, "pins and needles" sensations (paresthesias), and shooting pains.

They are most likely to occur after chronic exposure. Marked improvement of carpal tunnel syndrome has occurred among patients with aspartame disease after they avoid avoided aspartame products (Chapter VI-E).

Inflammation of the pancreas (pancreatitits)

"Pancreatitits was the probably basis for severe abdominal pain in some aspartame reactors (Bennett 1952) (Chapter IX-D).

Inflammation of the heart muscle (cardiomyopathy).

"A number of patients with aspartame disease complained of palpitations, rapid heart action and atypical chest pain (Chapter IX-C). Persons who smoke heavily and ingest much aspartame are probably at greater cardiovascular risk. (Cigarette smoke also may contain methyl alcohol.).

"Monte (1984) alluded to the case of a 21 year old man who worked as a material handler in the aspartame area of a plant that packaged this product. He was exposed to a fine dust of aspartame daily for seven months. The patient developed a dilated heart, and ventricular ectoy requiring quinidine. Other complaints included visual disturbances, headache, dizziness and severe depression.

At autopsy, an enlarged and dilated heart due to cardiomyopathy was found.

"The author has received reports of other persons working in a similara environment whose illnesses were attributed to inhaled aspartame. (Chapter XXVII-G).

Central Nervous System Involvement

"The cerebral effects of methanol contribute to the magnitude of neurologic and psychiatric manifestations in aspartame disease (Chapters III, V, VI and VII).

"Imaging studies of the brain in patients with methyl alcohol toxicity have revealed areas of presumed infarction (McLean 1980); Shwartz 1981). Methanol intoxication causes symmetrical necrosis and hemorrhage of the putamen.

"Marked reduction of both cerebral blood flow and cerebral blood flow and cerebral oxygen consumption have been documented during methanol poisoning.

"Observations concerning brain edema and vascular stasis after methanol exposure are also relevant to the neuropsychiatric reactions in aspartame disease.

* "Edema of the brain in methanol poisoning has been found in humans and animals (Menne 1938; Bennet 1953; Erlanson 1965; Rao 1977).

* "Rao et al (1977) noted significant alterations in brain water, sodium and potassium when methanol was administered to male rabbits and monkeys. Concomitant vascular stasis was evidence by colloidal carbon studies. These changes occurred in both acute and chronic studies. (With chronic administration, the concentration of blood methanol progressively increased after the third week, suggesting partial inhibition of methanol degradation.)

"Methanol-induced parkinsonism has been attributed to postsynaptic dysfunction, perhaps by interference with dopamine reuptake at nerve terminals. McLean et al (1980) reported two survivors of acute severe methanol intoxification who developed parkinsonism, dementia, other neurologic abnormalities including bilateral Babinski responses), and blindness due to optic atrophy.

"The National Institute for Occupational Safety and Health (NIOSH) includes methyl alcohol in Organic Solvent Neurotoxicity (Current Intelligence Bulletin Volume 48, March 31, 1987). The neuropsychiatric features of chronic toxicity from organic solvents range from a mild "organic affective syndrome" (characterized by fatigue, impaired memory, irritability, mild mood disturbances and difficulty in concentrating) to severe toxic encephalopathy with profound and generally irreversible dementia."

Dr. H. J. Roberts also discusses the fact that the methanol consumed in aspartame beverages could readily exceed 250 mg. daily, especially in hot weather or after exercise. This is 32 times the consumption limit for methanol recommended by the Environmental Protection Agency (EPA).

Methanol concentrations are likely to be higher when aspartame products have decomposed during exposure to heat or prolonged storage.

Traditional Herbal Remedies to help with Diabetes

For many years, before the attack on herbs began in earnest, many people were helped by a natural approach that supported the pancreas, adrenal glands, and the liver. One excellent herbal blend made from cedar berries, golden seal, uva ursi, cayenne, licorice root, and mullein has been used to correct both hyper and hypo glycemia, the Pancreas Tea. Working with this pancreas formula is a good and supportive herbal formula to support adrenal function. Many times the adrenal glands are over stressed in chronic dis-ease. Mullein, licorice, Siberian ginseng, gotu kola, hawthorne berries, lobelia, cayenne, and Ginger are found in this blend.

Mullein and Lobelia: the perfect glandular foods.

Siberian Ginseng: Successfully used in the Soviet Union to ease stress in everyday situations and tend endurance to athletes under great strain during training.

Gotu Kola: Known to help promote the stimulation of the brain and relieve fatigue when given in small amounts. Wonderful for the functioning of the pituitary in disorders of the adrenal system when used in conjunction with other herbs.

Hawthorn Berries: A celebrated cardiac tonic for many centuries. Under conditions of stress, the heart often "works overtime." Hawthorn berries can help in treatment of high or low blood pressure, tachycardia, and arrhythmia. It is also anti-spasmodic, sedative, and soothing to nerves, especially in nervous insomnia.

Cayenne: Nature's finest stimulant; source of calcium and vitamin A. Aids in circulation of blood which brings oxygen and other nutriments to cells in need of repair.

Ginger: A stimulant and a 'lead sheep' herb, bringing the other herbs in the formula into the abdominal area. Ginger differs from cayenne as a stimulant, in that the cayenne stimulates the heart, arteries, veins and then the capillaries. Ginger starts its stimulating effect in the capillary, flushing out the "constipated" capillary, driving these wastes into the veins for disposal.

Helping your liver and kidneys is the next part of this approach - Taking this herbal combination with parsley tea is a great help to your kidneys: juniper berries, parsley root, marshmallow root, golden seal, uva ursi, lobelia, ginger.

Creating Health Institute

Liver herbs that help - of course milk thistle, but blend these herbs for a good nutritional base to support your liver and gall bladder. I personally believe that gall bladder issues are common in people with diabetes. Barberry, wild yam, cramp bark, fennel seed, ginger, catnip, peppermint.

For many years I have been recommending safflower oil especially for use when neuromuscular health problems are involved, and with immune disorders. New information follows showing help for metabolic sensitivity, etc. A daily dose of safflower oil, a common cooking oil, for 16 weeks can improve such health measures as good cholesterol, blood sugar, insulin sensitivity and inflammation in obese postmenopausal women who have Type 2 diabetes, according to new research. Ohio State University (2011, March 21). A dose of safflower oil each day might help keep heart disease at bay.

ScienceDaily. Retrieved March 22, 2011, from http://www.sciencedaily.com/releases/2011/03/110321134629.htm

The fruit fly study and other studies seem to suggest that fat and consumption may not have the negative effect upon longevity and weight control that current thinking has portrayed them to have. In fact, the food pyramid with a heavy carbohydrate (often yeast based products) base may actually cause increased obesity and lessen the human life span. It is time to through conventional wisdom out the window, and take a look at the fact that individuals have gotten fatter with during the past twenty years not thinner.

During these same twenty years low fat and low protein diets have been touted as the way to a thinner healthier individual, sadly statistics indicate that this approach does not work.

B Vitamins - I have noticed that when I have adequate B vitamin levels I do not react to wheat. Many with diabetes suffer from low B vitamin levels and wheat allergy.

Chokecherry - An elephant never forgets ... two portions of aronia berries a day helps prevent memory loss. Constituents of high orac value fruits act as anti-inflammatories which reduce inflammatory states associated with chronic dis-ease like diabetes.

ARONIA BERRIES: These North American berries have three times the level of antioxidants found in blueberries.

Prevention is better than cure ... purple asparagus protects against diabetes Natural Health News: Asparagus, an olde cancer-fighting remedy A single serving of asparagus also provides 60 per cent of our recommended daily allowance of folate - a form of vitamin B9.

This reduces levels of amino acids which can cause cardiovascular disease and stroke. An anticancer food too. Did you know that asparagus is one of the best sources of folate (or folic acid)? Your body requires folate to replace all the cells lining your digestive tract every few days and all of your oxygen-carrying red blood cells every few months. Folate also helps repair all wounded, aging or damaged cells, helps to keep the cells of your heart and nervous system in top form, and maintains the normal metabolism of homocysteine into harmless compounds (high levels of homocysteine are a marker for increased risk of heart disease). Plus, folate is essential for reproductive health since it forms the protective cells covering the cervix and is necessary for the formation of sperm as well as every cell of a growing fetus inside a pregnant woman. One cup of cooked asparagus provides 66% of the daily value for folate

PURPLE ASPARAGUS: Eating this significantly increases the action of insulin, combating excess blood sugar and in the long-term helping to prevent the onset of diabetes.

Achieve metabolic balance: Eliminate toxins, maximize nutrition.

Getting back to vitamin B6 P5P is the bioactive form of vitamin B6 (pyridoxine). Big PhRMA has acted to "control" P5P so it is not available on the open market, except with prescription. I use this form and also take it in combination with B6 as in my work I have found that the two together boost utilization. When B6 levels are adequate atherosclerosis is unlikely to occur. Related to this is research that did look at utilization. The findings showed that the amino acid cysteine needed B6 to convert methionine to cystathione and on through the cycle to cysteine. It was found as well that most people in nutrient deficient states could not achieve this result. B6 and cysteine need each other and the efficient use of these nutrients help block the addictive nature of cravings because of low nutrient levels. This research supports the need to look to providing adequate nutition to achieve adequate nutrient levels of these key vitamins, minerals, and proteins (amino acids). An easy way to supplement your diet is to use organic nutritional yeast as it is an excellent source of all B vitamins, amino acids, and trace minerals.

Yes, B6 is needed in any conversion of amino acids or protein

CHI reported on this in 2004 - (Avandia) Rosiglitazone increased the risk of heart attack by 16%, heart failure by 23%, and death by 14%. Banned in Europe, not in US Banned diabetes drug alternative www.bbc.co.uk A drug to treat diabetes, Actos, would be a "sensible alternative" to one which was banned last year, say researchers. Actos now associated with bladder cancer.

Iodine Alternatives: Activated Charcoal, Rosemary tea, Thyme tea, Clay baths, Cook organic brown rice with red onion and dulse for heavy metal detox (cilantro isn't the best for heavy metal detox).

More about increase in obesity, heart disease, diabetes - and this makes sense. Now I find some one who has objected to the nonfat low fat diet like I have for decades. Carbohydrates, But Not Saturated Fats contribute To Heart Disease As reported by Melinda Moyer in Scientific American, the U.S. government has stated over the last thirty years that we should consume less saturated fat in our diet for the prevention of heart disease.

However, even though the percentage of daily calories from saturated fats have been reduced by many Americans since 1970, the obesity rate has more than doubled, diabetes has tripled and heart disease is still the biggest killer. She also sites almost two dozen studies that account for this rise and that is the increased consumption of processed carbohydrates. A study in the American Journal of Clinical Nutrition based on over three hundred thousand individuals followed over a period of five to twenty three years, reported that no association was found between the amount of saturated fat intake and the risk of heart disease. The past studies reporting the conventional wisdom that saturated fat is bad for the heart is based mostly upon extrapolations with little data to support it.

Further "total cholesterol" is not a great predictor of risk. Even though saturated fat may increase levels of LDL, they also increase HDL. Studies have shown that in groups consuming a low carbohydrate diet and who consumed the most saturated fat compared to low fat diets had the healthiest ratio of HDL to LDL cholesterol levels. Moyer, MW. Carbs Against Cardio.

More data that refined carbohydrates, not fats, threaten the heart. Sci. Amer. May, 2010. SiriTarino, PW, et al. Saturated fat, carbohydrate, and cardiovascular disease. Am. J. Clin. Nutr. 91, 3, 2010.

A related issue and one I have been education people about for a long time. This is a 2006 article. If you have a Rx for Metformin and no one told you about the B12 depletion then give them a piece of your mind! And demand B12 shots, s/b 2800 mcg daily at least for chronic disease.

Diabetic Drug Treatment Leads To B12 Deficiency

Metformin is a drug commonly used in the treatment of patients with type 2 diabetes. Common trade names include Glucophage XR, Riomet, Fortamet, Glumetza, Obimet, Dianben, Diaformin and Diabex.

The action is primarily through its suppression of hepatic glucose production. This drug is associated with contributing to B12 deficiency. A study of 155 diabetic patients found that B12 deficiency was significantly associated with dose and duration of metformin use. The authors of the study stated their results "underscore the need for monitoring subjects undergoing highdose and/or prolonged course metformin therapy." Published in Physician's First Watch October 11, 2006.

CHI publishes an opt in newsletter with a Diabetes focus. We do charge a one time $5 fee to subscribe to this list. Insulin Sensitivity and Magnesium has been a frequent topic as it has been validated that people with diabetes (PWD) are magnesium deficient, as is most of our population. Adequate intracellular levels of magnesium can prevent diabetes. And this is why at Natural Health News, our Top 10 rated BLOG, we give you both sides of the story. The 40 or so years of direct involvement in health care as a provider and our expertise in natural health gives you insight not available in fluff media, including CNN.

And consider that this is a reason why health care is ranked 37th in the US and most people do not trust it. It is not health care it is disease management and the patient pays the price.

Dr. John Ioannidis, a foremost expert on clinical trial methodology has identified various factors that, in one way or another, confound the integrity of medical research reports. He found that "as much as 90% of the published medical information that doctors rely on is flawed."

B12 and B9 help CAD (coronary artery disease) often found deficient in people with diabetes. More of an issue if using statin drugs as these drugs deplete many B vitamins needed to protect your heart.

Vitamin E - Nutritional Supplementation and Diabetes Mellitus - very important to be aware that many deficiencies can develop. Vitamin C, vitamin E, many herbs also are beneficial. Vitamin C can reverse diabetes, vitamin E prevents neuropathy and helps cardiovascular health.

Vitamin B12 - For many years I have been alerting people about the B12 deficiency caused by Metformin. A new study report just received today validates this. The longer you use this drug the more deficient you are. B12 is linked with healthy brain function and was a treatment used by doctors to treat dementia effectively. Lack of it can lead to anemia.

Iodine, The Usefulness of Iodine

Originally posted 4/11/08 Something already exists to help protect you from radiation, and it has been around for a very long time. It is often avoided in allopathic medicine these days because docs think you might want to take too much, which could be harmful. Seems that is a source: Natural Health News link: Full Article...

Don't forget that CHI has iodine products if you are not able to find what you need in your area. Find out more about radiation exposure on our veteran's page at simply4health.org

More about iodine here http://leaflady.org/usefulness_of_iodine.htm

Oatmeal, a healthy food, but make sure you use the best choice Are the various types of oatmeal nutritionally the same?

No, the different types of oatmeal are not at all the same in terms of nutrition. The very outermost portion of the oat-called the hull-is always removed before the oat is eaten. However, once the hull has been removed, there are several further processing steps that can be taken. Because these additional processing steps almost always serve to lower the nutritional value of the oats, I recommend the least number of additional processing steps to give yourself the best nourishment possible from your oats. The least processed forms for oats are oat groats and steel-cut oats. Oat groats consist of the hulled but unflattened and unchopped oat kernels. Steel-cut oats are the same as oat groats, except for being chopped with steel blades. Because they are the least processed, these two forms of oats are also the most nutritious.

Old-fashioned oats are chopped, steamed, and rolled to give them their flatter shape. Because they are more processed, they are less nourishing than oat groats or steel-cut oats. However, they are still better sources of nourishment than most quick-cooking oats or instant oatmeal. Quick and instant oatmeal usually have their oat bran-the layer of the grain that's just beneath the hull-removed. Many vitamins and much of the oat's fiber are contained within the bran, and so its removal is particularly problematic when it comes to nutritional value. Oat groats, steel-cut oats, and, to a slightly lesser extent, old-fashioned or rolled oats would be your best choices here, with quick and instant oatmeal usually being less nourishing due to further processing and the removal of their bran. Gluten free rolled oats is available from Montana now. We believe gluten free foods help reduce your risk of diabetes.

We recently tested Liquid Ionic Magnesium and found it to be very good. If using a supplement avoid aspartate form and oxide form when possible.

We offer hypoallergenic products approved by the Feingold Association, family owned since 1928, and other products.

The amino acid tyrosine is necessary for thyroid health, an indicator of the role of your thyroid in diabetes.

I follow a unique method of evaluating lab results developed at UCLA. My serum Mag range is 2-3, well above most lab test results. Magnesium is an essential ion for appropriate insulin sensitivity and insulin secretion. Serum magnesium levels should be routinely assessed in the subjects at high risk and in diabetic patients. If the hypomagnesemia is identified these subjects are candidates for magnesium supplementation.

Some good recipes but much of the other info is quite medical

Dil Se, Drive for Healthy Heart www.dilseindia.org

Method - Mix well all the ingredients together. Add in the dressing and mix well. Refrigerate till required. Serve chilled garnished with the chopped coriander.

Secondhand smoke linked to diabetes Secondhand smoke linked to diabetes | Reuters in.reuters.com

NEW YORK (Reuters Health) - Cigarette smoke is tied to a higher risk of type 2 diabetes, both for smokers and the people around them, a new study shows.And the more secondhand smoke people are exposed Passive smoking increases stillbirth risk http://www.bbc.co.uk/news/health-12711615

These chemicals can be a factor in diabetes http://leaflady.org/Grn_Lvg.htm Living on Earth: Chemical Review www.loe.org

Forty-five million different chemicals are commercially available around the world — and many of these chemicals go untested. Host Bruce Gellerman talks with Professor Patricia Hunt from Washington

State University who wrote a letter in the journal Science, calling for more stringent review of chemicals.

Cinnamon is actually good for many reasons. I like Kroeger Herbs Complete Concentrates Cinnamon caps because you get the herb AND the extract. One capsule following a meal will lower post-meal glucose elevation. The other supplements are fractionated. You can also use organic high oil content ground cinnamon which we offer. Most like the capsules.

Adding good information about vitamin B6 today. People with diabetes are 6 times more likely to suffer arteriosclerotic heart disease and stroke that those w/o DM. The key then is not cholesterol drugs but preventing the related complications that are not resolved by insulin, drugs, or questionable diet programs.

All of the vascular problems associated with diabetes are caused by nutritional deficiencies created by the diabetic process. An ecological and biological approach to this health problem addresses the issues of the 40 some nutrients needed along with $H2O$ and $O2$ and good body temperature. One example of this is the depletion of vitamin B12 caused by the drug Metformin.

All nutrients are important and amino acids, vitamins, minerals and enzymes all work together in various proportion in each person in a different formation unique to that individual.

One major study done decades ago showed that 100% or participants showed allergic reactions to specific foods and all had elevated blood sugar after ingesting the offending food AND vitamin B6 utilization deficiency. In the same group, over 86% showed deficient urine vitamin C levels. This showed that high blood sugar (HBS) caused severe depletion of vitamins B6 and C. 47% also sowed severe depletion of B9 (folic acid). Other nutrient deficiencies were believed to occur although not tested.

Another study was completed in Australia and found that there is a direct relationship between diabetes and B6 deficiency and that the B6 level was much lower than in non-diabetic people. They also found that B6 levels in people with diabetes (PWD) had even lower levels when cardiovascular problems were present.

Real Milk is Raw Milk 2011 UPDATE - March Only 2 deaths from raw milk, that was really cheese.

Sounds like Big Dairy is in control of your food choices at CDC. There's another related number that has been around much longer, and it's this: Between 1998 and 2008, there have been two deaths from raw milk source: Natural Health News link: Full Article...

Sit and Be Fit, an exercise plan for people who cannot stand Exercise Critical for PWD: The Benefits of Cardio Before Strength Training

Proper levels of GTF Chromium was proven in the 1960s to accomplish this, why another risky drug at high cost ? FDA accepts Bristol-Myers, AstraZeneca type 2 diabetes investigational compound NDA - Pharmaceutical

My colleague Dr Phil...Food allergy, IMHO is an issue in diabetes that is not even considered. Read what Dr Phil Bate says about the paleo diet and pulse testing for allergy. You'll learn lots! Caveman Diet & Pulse Testing for Allergies/Sensitivities

Is a cholesterol drug really helping your health? http://www.herballegacy.com/Cholesterol.pdf

Glycemic Index is good to know about, Glycemic Load data may be more helpful Decoding the glycemic index newhope360.com Learn how to interpret the glycemic index, and which carbs are the smartest dietary choices (hint: they're not all evil!).

Another source on Glycemic Index http://viewer.zmags.com/publication/547708e7#/547708e7/1

More on GL http://organicconnectmag.com/wp/2011/03/decoding-the-glycemic-index/

Dr Briffa is one of my fav natural MDs http://www.drbriffa.com/?s=glycemic+load&submit=Search

Patrick Holford http://www.facebook.com/%2Fpages%2FPatrick-Holford%2F116484061732127

From our website http://www.leaflady.org/G_index.htm

The Diabetes Fighting Tomato The Ultimate Diabetes-Fighting Fruit

It doesn't matter if you say "tom-ay-to" or "tom-ah-to," so long as you say, "yes" to eating them.

These juicy fruits (yes, tomatoes are fruits) are incredibly low in calories (just 22 per tomato!) and carbs (less than 5 grams each). What's more, they're rich in vitamin C, which helps protect the body from blood-sugar damage. They're also rich in lycopene, a nutrient that's a member of the beta-carotene family that has proven blood-sugar stabilizing effects.

Lycopene is also a powerful antioxidant. Men who eat tomatoes and tomato products such as tomato paste and tomato sauce at least twice a week lower their risk of prostate cancer by 24 to 36 percent!

There are also studies that have linked tomatoes to reduced risk of osteoporosis, asthma, and inflammation.

Tomatoes are so versatile, the opportunities to eat them are endless. Of all the veggies and fruits to incorporate into your diet, they are some of the easiest to use. Because lycopene is fat-soluble, it needs a little healthy fat to be absorbed into the body. That's an easy fix—tomatoes and olive oil go together famously. You can also serve them with nuts or avocados (other healthy fats). Here's more about the tomato http://www.leaflady.org/tomato.htm

US Health Care: Why We Rank Low. I have yet to see the AMA do anything that has stopped or changed these obstructions. What's wrong with U.S. Healthcare

Tulsi tea (a type of basil), very good tasting, helps diabetes. Tulsi www.horizonherb.com

Value in What You Read On Line

In 1956 researchers knew that chromium was very important in maintaining proper glucose metabolism. The dose used was 20-50 u of chromium /100 grams of weight. This immediately corrected glucose tolerance. These studies have been repeated successfully. This research proved that chromium was required for insulin utilization in glucose (sugar) metabolism. The only bioactive chromium was found to be the trivalent form, or what is known as GTF chromium.

In this form chromium is bound with two B3 (niacin) molecules and the amino acids cysteine, glycine and glutamine.

Taking insulin or glucose requires that chromium levels from liver stores increase within 30-120 minutes in non-diabetic people.

Sugar in foods depletes chromium. In diabetes, people excrete very high amounts of chromium via urine. And chromium exerts its action on insulin in tissues.

As you eat more sugar or take more insulin you continue to deplete chromium which leads to glucose intolerance and a need for more insulin. Rarely do you see any doctor telling a person with diabetes to take chromium, such as 5 PPM in drinking water which immediately reverses the equivalent of diabetes.

Carbohydrates other than sugar may also cause chromium depletion.

Using organic whole wheat flour supplies 175 mg of chromium in 100 grams of wheat. White flour supplies 23 mg of chromium.

Henry Schroeder MD said that the typical American diet was clearly designed to supply as little chromium as possible, BUT, to also cause urinary depletion of chromium, necessary for proper metabolism. The refining and processing of food is directly related to this problem.

In 1960, Dr Schroeder also showed that arteriosclerosis was a directly related problem to the lack of chromium and over dependence on processed foods. His results showed that without chromium, diabetes and elevated cholesterol was rampant.

My colleague, Gary Null, PhD, suggest up to 600 mg of chromium supplementation a day, or more.

Approximately 21 million Americans have diabetes, a condition characterized by abnormally high levels of glucose (sugar) in the blood. There are two forms of diabetes: type 1 and type 2. In people with type 1 diabetes, mild abnormalities in the retina begin to appear an average of seven years after the diabetes begins, but damage that threatens vision usually does not develop until much later.

In people with type 2 diabetes -- the more common type -- retinopathy may be present at the time of diagnosis or relatively soon afterward. This is because the onset of type 2 diabetes is gradual, and changes in the retina may have already taken place before the diabetes is even diagnosed. Here are the three progressive stages of diabetic retinopathy:

* Microaneurysms -- In the early, or nonproliferative, stages of diabetic retinopathy, blood vessels in the retina develop weak spots that bulge outward (microaneurysms) and may leak fluid and blood into the surrounding retinal tissue. These initial abnormalities usually cause no visual symptoms, and in many people the disease progresses no further. However, microaneurysms can lead to macular edema.

* Macular Edema -- Swelling around the macula (macular edema) caused by the leakage and accumulation of fluid can occur in people with diabetes. The swelling alters the position of the retina and causes blurred vision. Loss of vision is more pronounced when the center of the macula is affected.

* Proliferative Retinopathy -- This is the most dangerous form of diabetic retinopathy, characterized by neovascularization -- the growth of new blood vessels onto the back surface of the vitreous humor.

Acute loss of vision can occur when new blood vessels rupture and bleed into the vitreous humor or when these blood vessels lead to traction on the retina, causing it to detach from the back of the eye (retinal detachment).

Experts don't yet know exactly how high blood glucose levels cause diabetic retinopathy. One possibility involves a protein known as vascular endothelial growth factor (VEGF), which promotes the growth of new blood vessels in the eye and is secreted into the eye in response to damage caused by diabetes. Studies also suggest that elevated levels of cholesterol and triglycerides as well as high blood pressure can increase the risk of diabetic retinopathy. These conditions are more common in people with diabetes than in the general population.

Posted in Vision on January 21, 2011

Statin drugs increase incidence of cataract A cataract is an opacification (cloudiness) of the eye's normally clear crystalline lens. Cataracts can occur at any age, but they are most common later in life. In the United States, 75% of people over age 60 have some sign of cataracts. Now a study reported in the journal BMJ (Volume 340, page 2197) suggests that statins, the widely used class of cholesterol-lowering drugs, are associated with an increased risk of cataracts.

Investigators reviewed information from more than two million people in England and Wales, ages 30 to 84, in the QResearch medical database between 2002 and 2008. Of that group, 225,992 were new

users of one of the following statins: simvastatin (Zocor), atorvastatin (Lipitor), pravastatin (Pravachol), rosuvastatin (Crestor), or fluvastatin (Lescol).

The investigators found that statin use was associated with an increased risk of cataracts in both men and women. The risk of cataracts rose within one year of starting statin treatment, persisted during treatment, and then returned to normal within a year after discontinuing the statin.

Bottom line: This study was not designed to show whether statins could cause cataracts, but it does show an association between the two. These findings conflict with other recent studies that have found that statins may prevent cataract development. More studies are needed to provide a definitive answer. In the meantime, it's important to see your eye doctor regularly to monitor for cataracts and other eye diseases.

Posted in Vision on March 4, 2011

ASPARTAME AND SPLENDA INFORMATION If you have diabetes or know someone who does, please get educated.

"Zerose, Zevia or what ever you wish to call it, it...":

My boyfriend and I had thought we found the holy grail "HEALTHY SODA".....fast forward two weeks later we can MOST DEFINITELY attribute our painful gas and bloating/diarrhea to the soda.

We love the taste, but the pain is not worth it.

This is Truvia as well.

Aspartame causes an irregular heart rhythm and interacts with all cardiac medication. It damages the cardiac conduction system and causes sudden death. You can go to www.mpwhi.com and click on sudden cardiac deaqth and you will read a lot about cardiac problems.

A new study recently linked diet drinks with heart attacks and strokes.

As to your physician he should get the experts medical texts on aspartame in order to understand. The web sites are also full of articles . You can have your physician call me if you like, 770 242-2599. See below for the Aspartame Resource Guide which will gives you the names of books.

Aspartame Resource Guide

Aspartame medical text, Aspartame Disease: An Ignored Epidemic,www.sunsentpress.com by H. J.

Roberts, M.D., over 1000 pages He also has other books on aspartame and just published "A Manifesto for American Medicine"

Dr. Leonard Coldwell's Detox Formula: http://www.mpwhi.com/resources-coldwell.htm His new book is "The Only Answer to Cancer".

Detox formula: "What To Do If You Have Used Aspartame" by neurosurgeon Russell Blaylock, M.D., www.wnho.net/wtdaspartame.htm Dr. Blaylock is author of

Excitotoxins: The Taste That Kills, www.russellblaylockmd.com He has an excellent CD titled: "The Truth About Aspartame", www.atavistik.com All info is onhttp://www.mpwhi.com/blaylock_wellness_center.htm

Aspartame documentary: Sweet Misery: A Poisoned World, cori@soundandfury.tv

Aspartame Information List, you can subscribe on www.mpwhi.comscroll down to banners.

How to get aspartame out of your state: http://www.thenhf.com/press_releases/pr_24_feb_2009.html

Information on how aspartame blinds: http://www.mpwhi.com/nfb_aspartame_and_vision.htm

Safe Sweetener: Just Like Sugar, www.justlikesugarinc.om Can be found in places like Whole Foods.

Made of chicory and orange peel, Calcium and Vitamin C. Chicory has been used for 70 years to improve the health of diabetics. Dr. Russell Blaylock wrote in his newsletter, The Blaylock Wellness Report,www.russellblaylockmd.com "Finally a safe sweetener".

Aspartame Warning Flyer for distribution: http://www.mpwhi.com/warning_flyer_on_aspartame.htm

The Lethal Science of Splenda: http://www.wnho.net/splenda_chlorocarbon.htm

Studies have shown that sucralose can:

* Cause the thymus to shrink by as much as 40% (the thymus is your immune powerhouse - it produces T cells)

* Cause enlargement of the liver and kidneys

* Reduce growth rate as much as 20%

* Cause enlargement of the large bowel area

* Reduce the amount of good bacteria in the intestines by 50%

* Increase the pH level in the intestines (a risk factor for colon cancer)

* Contribute to weight gain

* Cause aborted pregnancy low fetal body weight

* Reduce red blood cell count

Particular warning to diabetics: Researchers found that diabetic patients using sucralose showed a statistically significant increase in glycosylated hemoglobin, a marker that is used to assess glycemic control in diabetic patients. According to the FDA, "increases in glycosolation in hemoglobin imply lessening of control of diabetes."

Here is how Splenda is made:
http://www.wnho.net/chemical_processing_of_splenda.htm

Ajinomoto just announced a new name for aspartame called AminoSweet. Be warned.

Web sites: www.mpwhi.com, www.dorway.com and www.wnho.net

Aspartame Toxicity Center, www.holisticmed.com/aspartame

Aspartame makes really good ant poison.

ASPARTAME We are non-profit and what we do is warn the world. We have Mission Possible operations in 50 states and 42 countries of the world that do nothing but warn people not to use aspartame. It is an addictive, excitoneurotoxic, carcinogenic, genetically engineered drug and adjuvant . MISSION POSSIBLE WORLD HEALTH INTERNATIONAL www.mpwhi.com Go to www.mpwhi.com and at the top of the web page you will see the FDA list of 92 symptoms they will admit to and notice seizures mentioned 5 times, different types of seizures. It also interacts with anti-seizure medication. Aspartame is a deadly poison and it also causes sudden cardiac death. Anyone with diabetes should avoid this and splenda.

Janumet FYI or sitagliptin, a genetically engineered pharmaceutical http://www.rxlist.com/januviadrug-patient.htm where you can read more about side effects

Black Box Warning for Janumet – LACTIC ACIDOSIS - lactic acidosis is a rare, but serious complication that can occur due to metformin accumulation. The risk increases with conditions such as sepsis, dehydration, excess alcohol intake, hepatic insufficiency, renal impairment, and acute congestive heart failure.

The onset is often subtle, accompanied only by nonspecific symptoms such as malaise, myalgias, respiratory distress, increasing somnolence, and nonspecific abdominal distress.

Laboratory abnormalities include low pH, increased anion gap and elevated blood lactate.

If acidosis is suspected, JANUMET1 should be discontinued and the patient hospitalized immediately.

[See WARNINGS AND PRECAUTIONS.]

Diabetes and Hearing Loss Is Diabetes Affecting Your Hearing?

It's long been known that diabetes can cause serious damage to your blood vessels. This is why diabetes is a leading cause of blindness, kidney failure, and heart disease in America. But did you know that the same type of diabetes-related blood-vessel damage can affect your ears, diminishing your ability to hear?

Diabetes can cause nerve damage that diminishes hearing. And some research suggests that diabetes can cause a shortage of a type of protein important to ear health. Add it up and people with diabetes are about twice as likely to experience hearing loss as people of the same age and background who don't have the disease. "Hearing loss may be an under-recognized complication of diabetes," the National Institutes of Health declared in a 2008 report.

Chances are, you are reading this thinking, "My hearing is just fine." But is it? Believe it or not, it's rarely obvious to you if you're losing your hearing. For most people, hearing loss happens very gradually; to them, the sounds of the world still seem plentiful and relatively clear, even if their hearing is in decline.

Loved ones and friends are often the first ones to notice your hearing loss, not you.

There are a lot of myths surrounding hearing loss. The biggest is that you have to be "older" to have it.

But most people with hearing loss are under 65 years old. And the percentage of younger people with hearing issues is getting larger, as modern audio technology and headphone use continues to increase.

Do you frequently ask others to repeat themselves? Are you constantly turning up the TV or radio volume? Do you have trouble following conversations in loud restaurants or big groups? Do you think that people are always mumbling? If you answer "yes" to more than one of these questions, you might want be screened for hearing loss.

People with diabetes should be diligent about getting routine hearing tests. At your next physical, ask your doctor to screen your hearing and even if you pass, share any concerns you may have. It can be easy to pass a hearing test in a quiet room but your day-to-day experiences are the real test. This is especially important for native people with diabetes because of the longstanding issues with hearing loss from childhood.

People with Diabetes (PWD) should have fewer carbs, more protein, increased exercise, weight management and a nutritional supplement program.

Steroids, like prednisone, can give you diabetes and many other illnesses. How steroids could give you diabetes www.dailymail.co.uk

They're drugs handed out by the million for asthma and arthritis. So why aren't we warned about a devastating side-effect?

Afternoon delight - think drink helps nourish adrenal glands and you: Sodium free V8 + nutritional yeast, or tomato. Also helps your thyroid, and gives you protein, B vitamins, minerals, energy. I have a similar recipe for hangover, helps to stop drinking too. My herbal formula to address drinking – Chalmer's Choice http://www.leaflady.org/newatCHI.htm

Habitual consumption of guarana may reduce metabolic disorders including hypertension, obesity and metabolic syndrome, according to new research. Guarana - Wikipedia, the free encyclopedia en.wikipedia.org

ˌɡaəˈɑː ˌeˈ ː Guarana (pronounced / w r n /, from the Portuguese pronunciation: [gwar na], Paullinia cupana (syn. P. crysan, P. sorbilis) is a climbing plant in the maple family, Sapindaceae, native to the Amazon basin and especially common in Brazil. Guarana features large leaves and clusters of flowers, a http://bit.ly/dUwYGj for more information

Probiotic could be "a promising tool" to treat ulcers. Some with H. pylori infection get diabetes which goes away when infection is gone. Probiotics help health overall. Probiotic could be "a promising tool" to treat ulcers: Study www.nutraingredients.com

Spanish researchers have described a strain of probiotic bacteria as a new "promising tool" in the treatment of ulcers caused by Helicobacter pylori in their report published in the latest edition of the journal Applied and Environmental Microbiology.

If taking statins you MUST take COQ10 - The potential benefits of co-enzyme Q10 (CoQ10) on LDL cholesterol levels may be linked to changes in the expression of specific genes, suggests a new study from Germany. http://www.nutraingredients.com/Research/CoQ10-may-benefit-cholesterol-via-geneexpression-Study/

COQ10 for many can help cholesterol better than statins w/o deadly risks

Many drink Green Tea but may not be aware that one study shows it can cause an increased risk of pancreatic cancer.

Many with DM use ALA or R-ALA. It has benefits but one risk is suppressed T3 thyroid hormone.

Occasional Chocolate May Support Diabetes Management.

This one is for Pokey @ Rosebud

By Jane Hart, MD

Occasional Chocolate May Support Diabetes Management : Main Image

Those who ate chocolate rich in cocoa solids and plant nutrients experienced improvements in cholesterol levels without significant changes in blood sugar

Research has shown that eating "heart-healthy" chocolate may protect against high blood pressure and ultimately heart disease. Now a study in Diabetes Medicine reports on the benefits of chocolate in people with type 2 diabetes—a population at great risk for heart disease – and found that those who ate chocolate rich in cocoa solids and plant nutrients experienced significant improvements in HDL

("good") cholesterol levels without significant changes in blood sugar control.

Chocolate raises good cholesterol

People with type 2 diabetes are typically told to avoid sweets, but research has shown that certain chocolate rich in cocoa solids and polyphenols (plant compounds that have health benefits) may affect blood sugar less than certain other foods such as potatoes or bread. This study looked at whether or not eating chocolate could help raise HDL cholesterol levels—another goal in preventing heart disease.

In this small study, 12 people with type 2 diabetes were randomly assigned to receive 45 grams of highpolyphenol chocolate (containing 85% cocoa solids) or low-polyphenol chocolate containing cocoa butter alone (containing no nonfat cocoa solids) once a day for 8 weeks. Participants continued their usual diabetes, high blood pressure, and lipid-lowering medications.

Results showed that people who ate the high-polyphenol chocolate had a significant increase in HDL cholesterol, and no significant change in weight or blood sugar control was seen in either group.

The study authors' point out: "This shows a potential for reduction in cardiovascular risk and combined with a lack of any deleterious effects on weight, markers of inflammation, insulin resistance or glycemic control. This appears to occur even in subjects treated with lipid-lowering therapies, indicating a beneficial additive effect through an alternate pathway."

Putting it in perspective

• More research is needed. While people with type 2 diabetes are often looking to expand day-to-day diet options, this small study alone probably isn't reason enough to start eating chocolate. A low-HDLcholesterol level is just one risk factor among many that may contribute to heart disease, and there are a number of ways to raise HDL including regular exercise. Further research is needed about the effects of chocolate on cardiac risk factors and particularly in people with diabetes.

• Talk with your doctor. A person with diabetes should always check with their doctor or dietitian before eating sweets such as chocolate, which can significantly raise blood sugar levels and lead to trouble. It is important to remember that the chocolate used in this study was designed specifically for study participants and not the same as the wide variety of chocolate found on most grocery store shelves, which is high in sugar and carbohydrates, low in nutrients, and can quickly raise blood sugar.

• Explore your options. If you have type 2 diabetes it is important to meet with a dietitian/nutritionist or diabetes educator who can help you explore day-to-day dietary options and most importantly, can help you learn to choose foods which will provide the most energy with the least effect on blood sugar, and minimize the risk for related chronic diseases, such as heart disease.

(Diabet Med 2010;27:1318–21)

Jane Hart, MD, board-certified in internal medicine, serves in a variety of professional roles including consultant, journalist, and educator at Case Medical School in Cleveland, Ohio.

I'll be adding more about the cholesterol myth as so many with diabetes get told to take the risky statin drugs. Pycnogenol to help protect kidneys in metabolic dis-ease.

Pycnogenol® Improves Kidney Function in Metabolic Syndrome Patients

Recent research on Pycnogenol®, French maritime pine bark extract, demonstrates kidney health benefits in metabolic syndrome patients. Published in Panminerva Medica, the study found that after supplementing with Pycnogenol®, patients experienced effective blood pressure control, reduced blood sugar, and further noticed lowered Body Mass index (BMI) due to weight loss. The results of the study demonstrate Pycnogenol®'s ability not only to control hypertension but also to restore kidney function in those impacted by metabolic syndrome. Additionally, patients not only demonstrated lower blood glucose levels, but also noticed significant weight loss during the six months of Pycnogenol® supplementation. This study reinforces previous studies that reveal Pycnogenol® is a natural solution for individuals with metabolic syndrome, particularly for kidney protection.

"This is the first study to our knowledge that has applied metabolomics to comprehensively assess the response to prolonged fasting in human volunteers," wrote the researchers.

Metabolic typing may bring dawn of personalised nutrition
www.nutraingredients.com

Personalized nutrition – seen by many as the future of nutrition – may take a step closer as scientists apply the metabolomics approach to identify individual metabolic 'types'.

CHI uses a system based on 80-100 years of research, many clients find it useful. Major use of this program led to a 1960s cure of liver & pancreatic cancer. Enzymes and right food choices does make a difference.

The Importance of Enzymes for Health, especially when you have diabetes "Nature's plan calls for food enzymes to help with digestion instead of forcing the body's digestive enzymes to carry the whole workload. If food enzymes do some of the work, according to the Law of Adaptive Secretion of Enzymes, the enzyme potential can allot less activity to digestive enzymes and have more to give to the hundreds of metabolic enzymes that run the body. If food enzymes did some of the work, the enzyme potential would not be facing bankruptcy, as it is now in the bodies of millions of people on the minus diet—food minus its enzymes. If the human organism must devote a large portion of its enzyme potential to making digestive enzymes, it spells trouble for the whole body because there is a strain on the production of metabolic enzymes and there may not be enough enzyme potential to go around. If humans take in more exogenous (outside) digestive enzymes, as nature ordained, the enzyme potential will not have to waste so much of its heritage digesting food. It can distribute more of this precious commodity to metabolic enzymes where it rightfully belongs."

-The late Dr. Edward Howell, M.D.

New science behind the importance of magnesium for metabolism, and more

Nutrigenomics shows benefit of magnesium's metabolic actions
www.nutraingredients.com

Magnesium's favorable effects on certain metabolic pathways is associated with changes in gene expression, says a new study that adds to our knowledge of nutrigenomics.

Four weeks of magnesium supplementation were associated with a decrease in levels of C-peptide, a marker of improved insulin sensitivity. The mineral was also linked to down-regulation of certain "genes related to metabolic and inflammatory pathways", according to findings published in the American Journal of Clinical Nutrition.

"These findings lend support to the hypothesis that dietary magnesium plays a beneficial role in the regulation of insulin and glucose homeostasis," wrote researchers led by Simin Liu, MD, ScD, Professor of Epidemiology and Medicine at the University of California, Los Angeles (UCLA).

Apples for health back in the news, read the same news from 16 years ago, and more from the 1930s/40s. Apples www.leaflady.org

Cancer Risk Higher if You have Diabetes Natural Health News: Cancer Risk Higher with Diabetes naturalhealthnews.blogspot.com

Vitamin E and Tocotrienols health promoting supplements for people with diabetes, lowers triglycerides, much more important than cholesterol.

First Aide tip for LW3: For sprained ankles Homeopathic arnica. Also for fast healing, an ace bandage soaked in apple cider vinegar, squeeze, apply loosely, cover in plastic bag. Overnight healing is possible.

More on benefits of vinegar here - It is a diabetes helper
http://www.leaflady.org/healing_with_vinegar.htm

Brown Rice helps diabetes.

Black beans are helpful to kidney health.

Natural Health News: Brown Rice: More than Low GL or High Fiber
naturalhealthnews.blogspot.com

I did not know about storing it in the fridge. Is this also true for rice bran oil? (Hard to find but great for cooking.)A nutritionist told me to stop eating white rice products because I may be pre-diabetic. I am allergic to wheat and many wheat-free products are high glycemic. She says that basmati...

This recipe for a breakfast cereal is helpful to keep blood sugar down-

Brown rice and sesame seeds.

Soak brown rice over night.

In the morning cook 1/2 cup rice in 1 and 1/2 cup water with a little salt.

Bring to a boil and then turn down to low heat, cover and cook 25 minutes.

When the rice is almost cooked add two tablespoons sesame seeds.

Makes 1 -2 servings.

Eat this with some cinnamon. Avoid using artificial sweetener, too much butter, or too much sugar.

Chopped apple is good to add a little sweet taste.

Backward Walking - This is a very helpful and restorative activity for your health. It helps too for brain injury (TBI, concussion, etc), improves memory and focus, more. Helps with knee injury, hamstring strain.

Physical Benefits of Backward Running and Walking
www.pyroenergen.com

Many people in Japan practice walking or running backward. In that way, it burns several times more calories than traditional way of jogging exercise.

More on backward walking
http://www.bodyresults.com/e2backwardswalking.asp

The latest Guidelines have moved away from a low-fat mantra, and focusing on healthier fats.

(US Dept of Health & Human Services Dietary Guidelines for Americans.

Dietary Guidelines for Americans | Health.gov (ODPHP)

The 2010 Dietary Guidelines for Americans provides evidence-based nutrition information and advice for people age 2 and older. This article from NPF continues - It's still recommended we consume 10% or fewer of total calories from saturated fat, which are found in animal foods and partially hydrogenated fats, but now we are urged to include plenty of mono- and polyunsaturated fats. To find these healthier fats, try fish, nuts, seeds, olives and olive oil, avocados, and liquid vegetable oils.

PLEASE NOTE - Liquid vegetable oils like soy and canola are the two that are highly propagandized.

Both are GMO for the most part, and Canola is toxic to your liver. Read labels, Canola oil is in almost everything, even "health" brands.

Natural Healing through Natural Health, www.leaflady.org, an honor to participate: **PROJECT PELION - An Adventure of Mountainous Proportion** 1981: International Year of the Disabled. People with diabetes were on this climb.

Understanding why sugar can be so deadly: GLYCATION

Does Sugar Caramelize the Heart?: www.cpmedical.net

When the general population discusses heart health, a lot of attention is paid to the effects of saturated fats on the cardiovascular system and on lipid levels. However, little attention is paid to the heart-harming consequences of consuming sugar. Yet, although saturated fat has taken the blame...

Sulfur helps minimize glycation. Pure MSM is a good source.

Nutrients for better eye health -

Oligomeric proanthocyanidins (OPCs) found in a variety of plants, fruits, and vegetables, are flavanols that offer strong antioxidant protection.

Natural Health News: Eye on ocular health in the computer era naturalhealthnews.blogspot.com

University of Maryland researchers suggest that carotenoids, particularly lycopene may protect the eye against oxidative damage and play a critical role in visual function. The identification of lycopene and a diverse range of dietary carotenoids in ocular tissues suggest that these carotenoids, …

Kale and Brussels sprouts contain phytonutrients that protect against free radicals–highly unstable molecules that affect cells and genetic material. They also stimulate the body's cleansing systems and are supportive in the healthy functioning of the eye.

Whole complexes of vitamins A, B and C are important for eye function. especially the retina.

Anthocyanin in bilberry fruit promotes vascular integrity and enhances microcircluation, enhancing blood flow to the eyes. Cayenne also helps this.

Ginkgo biloba extracts support healthy circulation and oxygen flow to the brain and eyes.

More from our web sitehttp://www.leaflady.org/vision.htm

More supporting evidence for eye nutrition - http://www.naturalproductsinsider.com/news/2011/02/nutrient-sensitivity-and-the-eye.aspx

February 2011

Insulin has three sulfur-containing cross-linkages and the insulin receptor has a tyrosine-kinase containing sulfur bond, which are the preferred targets for binding by mercury, lead and uranium.

Should any of these heavy metals attach to one of these three sulfur bonds it will interfere with the normal biological function of the insulin molecule.

Altern Med Rev. 2002 Feb;7(1):22-44. Parcell S

Sulfur in human nutrition and applications in medicine. . .

American Institute for Biosocial and Medical Research (AIBMR), Tacoma, WA, USA. steveparcell@attbi.com

Abstract

Because the role of elemental sulfur in human nutrition has not been studied extensively, it is the purpose of this article to emphasize the importance of this element in humans and discuss the therapeutic applications of sulfur compounds in medicine. Sulfur is the sixth most abundant macromineral in breast milk and the third most abundant mineral based on percentage of total body weight. The sulfur-containing amino acids (SAAs) are methionine, cysteine, cystine, homocysteine, homocystine, and taurine. Dietary SAA analysis and protein supplementation may be indicated for vegan athletes, children, or patients with HIV, because of an increased risk for SAA deficiency in these

Source groups. Methylsulfonylmethane (MSM), a volatile component in the sulfur cycle, is another source of sulfur found in the human diet. Increases in serum sulfate may explain some of the therapeutic effects of MSM, DMSO, and glucosamine sulfate. Organic sulfur, as SAAs, can be used to increase synthesis of S-adenosylmethionine (SAMe), glutathione (GSH), taurine, and N-acetylcysteine (NAC). MSM may be effective for the treatment of allergy, pain syndromes, athletic injuries, and bladder disorders. Other sulfur compounds such as SAMe, dimethylsulfoxide (DMSO), taurine, glucosamine or chondroitin sulfate, and reduced glutathione may also have clinical applications in the treatment of a number of conditions such as depression, fibromyalgia, arthritis, interstitial cystitis, athletic injuries, congestive heart

failure, diabetes, cancer, and AIDS. Dosages, mechanisms of action, and rationales for use are discussed. The low toxicological profiles of these sulfur compounds, combined with promising therapeutic effects, warrant continued human clinical trails.

PMID: 11896744 [PubMed - indexed for MEDLINE]

http://www.altmedrev.com/publications/7/1/22.pdf

Web site gone wild over dandelions for health. Get our organic extract.

http://www.leaflady.org/health_benefits_of_dandelions.htm

Uses for Dandelion Herbal Supplement

www.ehow.com

Dandelion populates many yards and fields. Though many consider it to be a pesky weed and many herbicides specifically target it, dandelion has a long history of use as a...

The Longest Walk 3/Reversing Diabetes 2011 Walk Across America begins 2/14/2011 on Betty Tuininga's. twitwall.com

Arriving in Washington, DC on July 8, 2011 (In less than 6 months) we will of embarked on another historic journey an event so great and much needed for all of America! THE LONGEST WALK 3 – REVERSING DIABETES.

herbalYODA Says | Internet Radio | Blog Talk Radio
www.blogtalkradio.com

Health & Natural Health Education and Advocacy, simply4health –
DETOX

Natural Health News: Two Thumbs Up for Daily Multiple
naturalhealthnews.blogspot.com

Diabetes 1 - Could it be allergy? Surely there is something to this! Even
Type 2. Think about it!

The Heart Scan Blog: Why is type 1 diabetes on the rise?
www.heartscanblog.org

Type 1 diabetes, also called "childhood" or "insulin-dependent"
diabetes, is on the rise. Type 2 diabetes, or "adult," diabetes, is also
sharply escalating. But the causes for this are easy-to-identify:
overconsumption of carbohydrates and resultant weight gain/obesity,
inactivity, as well as genet..

Vaccines also are a contributing factor for children, especially the
Hepatitis jab.

While controversial during his life, because he had unconventional
views, Harrower was a founder of endocrinology and believed diabetes
was a thyroid problem. His work was quite effective for many.

INFH :: International Foundation for Nutrition and Health
www.ifnh.org

INFH::Dr. Harrower's original text on the endocrine system was a
pioneering breakthrough for endocrinologist/organotherapist during
the first half of the 20th century

Gallbladder health is important to people with diabetes, 2009
study showing that Gallbladder health is important to people with
diabetes, it produces insulin

We have effective gall bladder health herbs and other treatment remedies. Do not lose it to a surgeon's knife. And fyi, fluoride drugs can cause sluggishness in the GB. So much more...

Australian researchers recently conducted a review of a number of studies and found there was a strong association between enteroviruses and the development of type 1 diabetes. In fact, children with diabetes were 10 times more likely to have had an enterovirus infection than children without the disease!
http://www.doctorshealthpress.com/diabetes#ixzz1EiDbjEur

Cold Virus Could Cause Onset of Type 1 Diabetes | Free Health Advice and Articles - Doctors Health P www.doctorshealthpress.com

A cold-like virus may be responsible for triggering the onset of type 1 diabetes.

Using full spectrum enzymes, amino acid compounds, Bicarbonate of soda (NAHCO3) with meals helps stave off after-meal hyperglycemia and side-effects of this reaction.

What heart and circulation problems can you get with diabetes?

Here is the mainstream outlook link. Check back as I add the natural information you need to protect your health.

http://www.consumerreports.org/health/conditions-and-treatments/heart-and-circulation-problemsin/

www.consumerreports.org

Exercise before eating is a whole different story.

When Is the Best Time to Exercise? www.thatsfit.com

Despite eating a horrible, weight gain-inducing diet, no weight gain. Group's insulin sensitivity remained high, the bad diet did not make the group insulin resistant. "This study for the first time shows that fasted (empty stomach) training is more potent than fed training to facilitate adaptations in muscle and to improve glucose tolerance and insulin sensitivity," said the study's authors.

Natural Health News is our main blog, an outgrowth of a net radio program we started at the end of the 90s. We are syndicated in at least 80 locations.

Natural Health News naturalhealthnews.blogspot.com

leaflady.org went online in 1991, our main domain

Natural Healing through Natural Health www.leaflady.org

An honor to participate PROJECT PELION - An Adventure of Mountainous Proportion1981: International Year of the Disabled People with Diabetes participated in Pelion

The Oake Centre for natural health education is our education and publishing group The Oake Centre simply4health.org

"I have learned more from your programs than from any other presentations I have attended." J.A., University of Idaho

Wound care help, when you do not have raw honey

Avocado Oils Fare Well in Wound Healing
www.insidecosmeceuticals.com

An oldie but hey, it's a goodie: In 2008, researchers in the West Indies wanted to know Persea Americana's (aka the avocado) fared on healing wounds.

Omega 3 does prevent retinopathy, and is very effective in the prevention of cardiovascular disease, inhibits blood clots, lowers cholesterol and triglycerides. Use marine oil sources. Vitamin B6 plays a part, more on this to come.

High or low amounts of fats or carbs are not atherogenic when enough supportive nutrients are present, start with B6. Focus on nutrient ratios in ref 'food categories'.

B complex source naturally, trace minerals, amino acids: Original hospital based trial showed reversal of gangrene, lowered blood sugar.

BioSUPPLEMENTE www.leaflady.org

Amino acid cysteine helps with B6 conversion to active form, p-5-p (Big PhRMA doesn't want you to have either form of this vitamin).

Dandelion root, chicory, cinnamon - all help keep blood sugar balanced.

Just Like Sugar if you like it sweet (made with chicory, no chemicals)

Dandelion Root Coffee (Serves 2-4)

4 cups water

2 tablespoons roasted dandelion root

2 tablespoons roasted chicory root

1 cinnamon stick

Place water, dandelion root, chicory root and cinnamon stick in a pot.

Bring to a boil, then reduce heat to simmer for 5 minutes.

Pour coffee through a small mesh strainer into cups and serve.

Vitamin D-fortified yoghurt improves weight and blood sugar control in diabetics | Dr Briffa's Blog www.drbriffa.com

Previously in this blog I have covered some of the evidence linking vitamin D with positive health outcomes, including a reduced risk of cardiovascular disease

Dr Briffa is one thinking doctor. This is good as using yoghurt (2% or higher) supplies protein, fat, and calcium - some of the factors needed to work with vit D effectively. It is easy to make your own but Nancy's or Zoi are good bgh free choices, PLAIN is best.

Here's more about yoghurt http://www.leaflady.org/yoghurt.htm

Researchers recommend greater intake of vitamin D to lower the risk of serious diseases, including diabetes (helps with reversing-preventing Type 1 http://www.leaflady.org/DHealth.htm

Researchers recommend greater intake of vitamin D to lower the risk of serious diseases - Life Extension www.lef.org

Cedric Garland, DrPH of the University of California, San Diego School of Medicine and his colleagues recently revealed that significantly higher amounts of vitamin D than what are currently recommended are needed to raise levels to those that help prevent breast cancer, type 1 diabetes and other...

Studies have made the link between diet-soda consumption and the risk of metabolic syndrome and diabetes. The Northern Manhattan Study is the first to show association between diet drinks and hard vascular-disease end points, according to Dr Larry Goldstein (Duke University Stroke Center).

Diet soda heightens vascular event risk in cohort study www.theheart.org

The latest developments in cardiology and cardiovascular research, including heartwire news and commentary by some of the world's top cardiologists.

Aspartame has always been known to cause diabetes and heart disease, Splenda may do the same as it calcifies kidneys. Just Like Sugar (inc dot com) SAFE sweetener for people with diabetes, made from vitamin C, extract of orange peel, and chicory

CHI extends its thanks to Jon Gabriel for the donation to our community library program.

The Anti Diet Book - The Gabriel Method - Lose Weight Without Dieting

www.gabrielmethod.com

I lost 113 pounds (51 kilos) in about six months and I've kept it off now for over a year. Also my blood

sugar levels went from a dangerously high 19 down to 6. I'm now within the normal range. They say I still have diabetes but I don't think so.

It is generally thought, from an orthomolecular (nutritional) perspective, that **Vitamin C can help to prevent or reverse Diabetes**. The dose for this therapy is 10 GRAMS daily.

It is best to titrate it by building slowly to this dose level. Contact us for the Vitamin C Flush that can be done as a prophylactic treatment at home. Clearly IV vitamin C, now under attack by the FDA, is a superior form of this therapy. Doses can be as high as 100,000 mg or more. Hep C and many cancers respond to this therapy as well. Vitamin C does not cause kidney stones and in many cases will break them down.

A good web site for nutrition information, health promoting recipes

The World's Healthiest Foods www.whfoods.org

This is the health promoting Food Pyramid that was axed in favor of Big AGs unhealthy one USDA wants you to follow

Natural Health News: Leading to Weightiness; Light on what happened to the healthy pyramid www.naturalhealthnews.blogspot.com

This is a many decades long well tested food plan that will reverse unbalanced biochemistry and improve health

INFH :: International Foundation for Nutrition and Health
www.ifnh.org

INFH::Dr. Melvin Page was one of the Pioneers in nutrition during the last century, his work in diet and lifestyle has been copied by many present-day practitioners. Dr. Page was the first to understand and perpetuate the significance of the calcium and phosphorus ratio.

Information on the risks of using Splenda, aspartame, neotame, acesulfame K, new ones like Truvia, Zevia, Purevia, etc. These make diabetes worse. We like the safe and natural sweetener Just Like Sugar.

MISSION POSSIBLE WORLD HEALTH INTERNATIONAL
www.mpwhi.com

Mark Gold has a good web site with more information
http://www.holisticmed.com/aspartame/

Lantus insulin is a genetically engineered insulin. One of the side effects is cancer.

You can always read the clinical data about drugs at rxlist.com, skip the patient info as it doesn't give you the ammunition to protect your health.

If you are taking multiple drugs you can do a drug interaction profile at drugs.com. The information gives you a good place to start a talk with your doctor as many of the interactions cause you to impair your health.

The importance of Balanced Blood Sugar

This article makes a very good point. The more stable and the more balanced blood sugar levels are the less problems ensue.

It is better to test more often and the newer meters encourage this although I know the strips are expensive. Once daily is just not enough and this is often what is suggested.

A capsule of Complete Concentrate Cinnamon does help keep your blood sugar down following meals.

Of course this is not new information, and it applies also to Type 2.

I would also say that the A1C may not be the very best way to measure this as I believe it is more or less an actuarial type test, with much too much focus placed on its use.

I would rather see much more frequent testing on a daily basis well beyond the one or twice a day metering.

Of course what you won't see in similar articles are the recommendations that neuropathy, retinopathy and kidney problems may all be prevented with adequate intake of vitamin E and C or some other nutrients in therapeutic doses along with a food plan, like the one we use in our work, that promotes balancing biochemistry.

Diabetes: Just Information and Daily Tips

I do not believe in making everyone with diabetes take statin drugs to lower cholesterol and I will write more about that later.

Stable blood sugar curbs diabetes complications By Martha Kerr Martha Kerr Fri Nov 21, 2:24 pm ET

NEW YORK (Reuters Health) – In people with type 1 diabetes, adequate control of blood sugar over the long haul helps reduce the risk of diabetes- related eye and kidney disease, new data suggest.

The findings stem from a look at 1,441 type 1 diabetic patients followed for roughly 9 years as part of the pivotal Diabetes Control and Complications Trial (DCCT).

By analyzing hemoglobin A1C levels over time -- a standard indicator of long-term blood sugar control the researchers observed that increasing variability in hemoglobin A1C heightens the risk of new or worsening diabetic retinopathy (damage to the retina) and diabetic kidney disease.

Specifically, for every 1 percent increase in hemoglobin A1C, they found that the risk of retinopathy increased more than twofold and the risk of diabetic kidney disease increased nearly twofold.

The findings suggest that the long-term stability of blood sugar, and not just the average blood sugar control, predict the risk of these complications, study investigator Dr. Eric S. Kilpatrick of Hull Royal Infirmary in Hull, England, noted in an interview with Reuters Health.

"It is probably another reason to aim for stable good glycemic control rather than only good glycemic control," Kilpatrick said.

However, blood sugar management "is only part of the story," he added. It is as important, he said, to ensure that blood pressure and cholesterol levels are "tightly controlled" in order to reduce the complications of diabetes.

SOURCE: Diabetes Care, November 2008.

Health will be better and there will be less disease on the rez when commodity foods are truly healthy.

Home urine test measures insulin production in diabetes
http://www.sciencedaily.com/releases/201...

A simple home urine test has been developed which can measure if patients with type 1 and type 2 diabetes are producing their own insulin. The urine test replaces multiple blood tests in hospital and can be sent by post as it is stable for up to three days at room temperature.

http://www.sciencedaily.com/releases/201

www.sciencedaily.com

http://www.sciencedaily.com/releases/2011/02/110224103240.htm

Fatty liver may herald impending Type 2 diabetes

Individuals with fatty liver were five times more likely to develop Type 2 diabetes than those without fatty liver. This higher risk seemed to occur regardless of the patient's fasting insulin levels, which were used as a marker of insulin resistance. Milk Thistle helps reduce or eliminate fatty liver.

Fatty liver may herald impending Type 2 diabetes
www.sciencedaily.com

Individuals with fatty liver were five times more likely to develop Type 2 diabetes than those without fatty liver. This higher risk seemed to occur regardless of the patient's fasting insulin levels, which were used as a marker of insulin resistance.

Here are two pages with information about the polluting effects of electromagnetic fields from cell phones et al. This is a pollutant that can affect people with diabetes, vision, heart, more. This one is about

the towers
http://blakelevitt.com/cell_towers__wireless_convenience__or_envir
onmental_hazard__proceedings_of_the___28525.htm

Electromagnetic Fields: A Consumers Guide to the Issues and How to
Protect Ourselves - B. Blake Levitt www.blakelevitt.com

Delta Dental and the Pew Foundation are funding this mandatory
fluoridation campaign using grants.

Arkansas getting mandatory fluoridation. More forced medication w/o
your consent. http://www.fluoridealert.org/

Both **aspartame and fluoride interfere with vaccines**, just be aware.

In today's news from Rodale Press they included an article about fats.
Here's an article I wrote several years ago when the Moscow ID
newsletter editor refused me my member right to contribute to the
newsletter. He opposed butter but he never would understand the
health benefit of saturated fat.

Fat Facts

www.leaflady.org

Natural Nutrition the foundation of health & healing - Fat Facts

It is important to know that the current push for "plant sterols"
encourages you to rely on soy and canola oils which are most likely
GMO sources. Canola oil, as I mention in my article, is toxic to your
liver.

This post from my blog explains more about the risk of soy and canola
oil

http://naturalhealthnews.blogspot.com/2008/07/canola-and-soy-oil-
not-worth-risk.html

Another point to consider is that there is a European study that shows that ALA can cause suppression of T3. Other issues are the inability to convert DHA to EPA, and I have more to write on this. This has to do mainly with plant based oils.

Artificial Sweeteners - independent scientific peer reviewed research honestly trying to find the truth showing that, "If you want to get fat NutraSweet is where its at". Aspartame Makes You Fatter: http://www.mpwhi.com/aspartame_makes_you_fatter.htm

Remember that aspartame changes brain chemistry, and as Dr. Richard Wurtman's affidavit says in the congressional record, it makes you crave carbohydrates. The congressional record is on a banner on www.mpwhi.com

Dr. Ralph Walton explains weight gain from aspartame this way:

Food seeking behavior and satiety are driven by an area of the brain known as the hypothalamus.

Stimulation of the medial hypothalamus in a laboratory rat leads to eating. Stimulation of the lateral hypothalamus leads to satiety and cessation of eating. Placing a lesion in the lateral hypothalamus produces an obese rat. The lateral hypothalamus is drive by serotonin. There are many papers in the current literature demonstrating that antidepressants which increase serotonin (but not antidepressants which act on other neurotransmitters) are useful in treating binge eating disorders. I believe that consuming large amounts of aspartame decreases the availability of serotonin and is thus analogous to placing a lesion in the lateral hypothalamus. Although much of this work is recent, clinical suggestions that aspartame can lead to a paradoxical increased appetite data back to Blunder's work in 1986.

An evolving view in modern psychiatry is that although depression, obsessive compulsive disorder, panic disorder, impulse control disorders and eating disorders have historically been viewed as separate entities, in fact, they should be viewed as a continuum of disorders all involving some degree of dysregulation of serotonin. I believe that at this time there is overwhelming evidence that aspartame contributes to this dysregulation.

Food scented products may play role in obesity epidemic:

Study http://www.foodnavigator.com/Science-Nutrition/Food-scented-products-may-play-role-inobesity-epidemic-Study/?c=v1rstJo1ERy1HtFoNY27PA%3D

%3D&utm_source=newsletter_daily&utm_medium=email&utm_campaign=Newsletter%2BDaily

From The Longest Walk 3 web site http://lw3.internettechnologyservice.net/ with many thanks to Evans Craig

About Dr Gayle - Supporting LW3 through my nonprofit health education organization, CHI (see the Diabetes Diary on FB, CHI-Creating Health Institute). We focus on natural health education, products and services. Celebrating 50+ blending science with the natural healing arts. I am Choctaw (MS) on my mother's side, Chickasaw with a little Eastern Cherokee and Powhatan on my father's side. I am also descended from people in Scotland and England. Some of my family were founders of the US and served in the early government of this county. I worked as a tribal health director and consultant, and economic development. In the mid-90s I taught a program on Natural Healing for Diabetes for a number of Western Tribes and organizations. I am a nurse practitioner by education and considered to be an expert in natural health. You can learn more at my main domain, www.leaflady.org

Food combination makes flexible arteries

Posted on June 20, 2011 by Dr Gayle

Simply combining about 3-4 tablespoons of plain applesauce with the same amount of plain fat containing yoghurt and a dash of cinnamon you can be on your way to healthy arteries that are flexible and begin to hold less plaque/cholesterol. Other anti-cholesterol … Continue reading

Posted in Foods, **Tip of the day**, diabetes, nutrition

Tagged applesauce, arteries, cholesterol, DVT, herbs, plaque, supplements, vitamin E, yoghurt

Some important thoughts

Posted on June 20, 2011 by Dr Gayle

Poor detoxification may promote inflammation and losses in energy production resulting in health challenges, especially for people with diabetes (PWD). Inflammation particularly, and energy loss, further impair the ability of your liver to help in detoxification. Many natural substances are … Continue reading

Posted in Foods, Tip of the day, diabetes, nutrition, walk |

Healthy Breakfast Lowers Blood Sugar

Posted on June 20, 2011 by Dr Gayle

Over the years that I have worked in health and nutrition I have found that people with diabetes (PWD) do very well with this recipe. You will need Short Grain Brown Rice, organic is best, and sesame seeds. Soak one … Continue reading

Posted in Foods, Tip of the day, diabetes, nutrition, walk |

Diabetes Tip of the Day – Myth: Low-Calories Foods Help You Lose Weight

Posted on June 14, 2011 by Dr Gayle

Not always Processed low-calorie foods can be weak allies in the weight-loss war. Take sugar-free foods. Omitting sugar is perhaps the easiest way to cut calories. But food manufacturers generally replace those sugars with calorie-free sweeteners, such as sucralose (Splenda) ... Continue reading

Posted in Foods, Tip of the day, diabetes, nutrition, walk | Tagged diabetes, Diabetes Tip, Splenda |

Diabetes Tip of the Day – Phosphates in soft drink pose health hazards

Posted on June 9, 2011 by Dr Gayle

This contributes to osteoporosis as well – Phosphates in soft drink pose health hazards Researchers at the Harvard University used mice to assess the health effects of excess phosphates (a form of phosphorus), one of the ingredients in soft drinks. Large amounts of ... Continue reading

Posted in Foods, Tip of the day, diabetes, news, nutrition |

Diabetes Tip – A Massage Technique

Posted on April 18, 2011 by Dr Gayle

Circulation issues are critical for people with diabetes (PWD). One suggestion we offer frequently at CHI is to massage with sesame seed oil. Used commonly in Ayurveda and Oriental medicine, sesame seed oil offer healing properties for neuropathy. It helps ... Continue reading

Posted in Tip of the day, diabetes, walk |

Diabetes TIP – Fats

Posted on April 17, 2011 by Dr Gayle

Most people are being told that it is better for people with diabetes to use certain products like the newer type margarine in place of other sources of fat. The problem with these so called "safe" sources, generally referred to … Continue reading

Posted in Foods, Tip of the day, diabetes, nutrition |

Diabetes TIP – Aspartame

Posted on April 16, 2011 by Dr Gayle

Learn about aspartame, protect your health. Continue reading

Posted in Tip of the day, diabetes, nutrition |

Diabetes TIP – Modified Stevia

Posted on April 14, 2011 by Dr Gayle

I also support using stevia however it has to be the pure type or pure extracts (preferably not sourced from China because of product contamination issues). The new "manufactured" types of 'stevia' are really not just stevia. DO NOT CONFUSE … Continue reading

Posted in Tip of the day, diabetes, nutrition |

Diabetes TIP – Sucralose

Posted on April 8, 2011 by Dr Gayle

Sucralose is very damaging for people who have diabetes because it can lead to kidney calcification.

It causes seizures, headache, shrinkage of the thymus (part of your immune system) and more. It is NOT inert so it absorbs and leads to obesity. … Continue reading

Posted in Coordinator, National Diabetes Summit, Tip of the day, diabetes

Why I Advise Against Margarine - This is from my blog - http://naturalhealthnews.blogspot.com/2010/09/margarine-not-heart-healthy.html

from my web site - http://www.leaflady.org/fatfacts1.htm

from Leaflady.org

Diabetic Health where you will find many health related articles and information.

http://www.leaflady.org/Diabetic_Health.htm

Gayle Eversole

DIABETES E LIST

How to use Vitamin C to fight inflammation and Diabetes

You can do this same process with capsules or tablets. Vitamin C is an excellent vitamin to help fight diabetes.

http://www.perque.com/pdfs/Pt_Ascorbate_Slush_FIN.pdf

Aspartame is Dangerous: Carcinogenic!

Article reference:
http://www.laleva.org/eng/2006/05/aspartames_extreme_and_highly _fatal_carcinognesis.html

Aspartame is extreme, and highly fatal: Carcinogenesis!

I am one of the only few "Nutra Sweet Dissidents" to ever see the first (original) pre-marketing Aspartame toxicity studies. It has to be strongly emphasized! These first studies were done at only 1/1000th the legally required Aspartame dosage levels. (And for only sixty days!) The law specifies that one hundred times the "greatest possible maximum human consumption" must always be used in premarketing testing of animals. This law is entirely conservative, because it only allows for only a ten fold species to species variation of effect, and only a ten fold variation of individual effect within a given species:

In order to protect all humans who may ever ingest a given chemical! Only 3 cans of pop per day (level) scaled down the weight of each given animal species, was ever used, in spite of the thousands of ways Aspartame is presently dosed into us, even being "sneaked" in with yogurts, chewing gums, etc! (The FDA recently got a law enacted that "ASPARTAME" does not now even have to be at all mentioned on the product label itself!)

The phenylalanine isolate poisoning from Aspartame is exemplary of why this legally mandated testing standard, (even if followed,) is inadequate protection for human beings. PKU (phenylketonuria) is a human enzyme deficiency, leading to severe brain damage even if even a small amount of a balanced mix of proteins containing significant phenylalanine content is consumed! Moreover, all the tested animals metabolize phenylalanine outside the brain, while the human being metabolizes it inside the brain, and at its brain enzyme sites, with extreme damages resulting, (even in non PKU "normal" humans) from the bolus of Phenylalanine isolate obtained from a single can of Aspartame pop!

Both concepts are inadequate in the case of Aspartame because:

1. Aspartame is a highly synergized methyl alcohol poisoning, and all the test animals used have the proper enzyme channels to harmlessly break down methanol without processing it through the Methanol>formaldehyde>formic acid>carbon monoxide toxic axis. This entire toxic axis is the only way methanol, from Aspartame, can be at all metabolized in humans. The "hangover" after drinking alcoholic beverages, (which contain only small traces of methanol,) is a small example of this toxicity, (even though the ethyl alcohol itself, is a specific, and the most highly effective antidote known, for methyl alcohol toxicity.)

"Excitotoxins" also markedly increase the severity of their poisonings, as the two indicated factors of greater molecule size, and other incorporated toxic chemistries increase in their molecular makeup!

Moreover in methyl esters like Aspartame, the larger the ester, and the more highly toxic its other components, the far worse will be the poisoning from each methyl ester. Aspartame maximizes these two extreme toxicities!

2. Because the Aspartic acid is a dicarboxylic amino acid, (and therefore a powerful neural excitotoxin!) Aspartame then will also form its own diketopiperazine entity while sitting in solution, or even while being digested. This DKP form is an extremely far more highly chemically

reactive, and an even far greater and stronger polymerization agent, than the parent chemical in every case. DKPs therefore, are the major substrate class used in synthesizing plastics! The DKP form of Aspartame was (in even that minuscule dose, and for only 60 days) found to be number one 10/5/2010 La Leva di Archimede (ENG): Aspartam...laleva.org/.../aspartames_extreme_and... 1/2 chemical ever identified to cause brain cancers in rats!

(Even when the other chemicals tested were used at maximal dosages, and over lifetime test periods, in the animals tested.) Just 1/1000th the legally mandated dose of Aspartame, ingested for only 60 days, caused the highest incidence of brain tumor in rats, that any chemical ever tested at any dose, ever caused!

The Aspartame "dicarboxlic amino acid neural excito toxicity" is also molecularly maximized, when given the two factors entioned above, (which also maximize the methyl alcohol toxic axis toxicity.)

Medically well known examples of the extreme damage from these two factors and chemical classes, are "Guam Parkinson disease," and "Prince Edward Island shell fish: Domoic Acid" poisoning, both of which have caused extreme neurological disease epidemics in Guam (And all around the World's Oceans), and Prince Edward Island, with lifelong neural sequelae, and also additional disease generations, occurring in those epidemic's victims!(Just as Aspartame also always does!)

For a clearer presentation of the even greater picture of Aspartame's extreme toxicity, Plz get Ch 7 of "Sweet Mystery in The Present Darkness: What Ever Happened to We Scientists Who First Spoke Out

Against Aspartame?" from wnho.net,www.aspartame.ca, or dorway! (It is freely available, for free!)

Billions of Victims is also "free" on those sites!

While I was driving cab in Denver: Upon hearing this, one of my fares screamed out: "Doc! You are sure right! Within a year of the time we started drinking Aspartame pop, three of my immediate family members experienced brain tumors, even though there had never before even been a single brain tumor in our entire known family tree. Moreover, all three then were dead within the year following, in spite of all which medicine, surgery, and radiation had to offer them!" (This is because Aspartame so damages and defocus es the entire immune system!) The first six months after they put "Nutra Sweet" into our "diet" pop and soft drinks, the US brain cancer occurrence rate jumped 10%, and the US diabetes "new case" rate 30%!

In those first low dose Aspartame: FDA pre-marketing studies the infant monkeys ONLY showed up with a 100% incidence of Grand Maul epilepsy! Those human subjects then tested at only "three cans of Aspartame pop" level per day for just sixty days, also showed an immediate 250% increase of "all physical complaint" incidence. Two of the sixty people used as Aspartame test subjects, then immediately developed highly malignant cancers: One Breast carcinoma, and One Bone sarcoma.

Both test subjects were dead within the year following, in spite of all which medicine, surgery and radiation had to offer them! The Food and Drug Death Association (FDA) comment: "Well, that's all just insignificant!" When they then went ahead and marketed Aspartame under the influence of Reagan, Rumsfeld, and Dr Arthur Hull Hayes! (Hayes refused, but was, at that time, BLACKMAILED into approving Aspartame, by godfather Rumsfeld!) These names, along with the Bushes, who are the primal New World Order force, amongst all this human "Aspartame devastation" should live in Infamy!

Sincerely, James D. Bowen MD

Posted by Archimede on May 22, 2006 11:40 AM | Permalink

10/5/2010 La Leva di Archimede (ENG): Aspartam…laleva.org/
…/aspartames_extreme_and… 2/2

More information on aspartame on www.mpwhi.com,
www.dorway.com, andwww.wnho.net

Aspartame Toxicity Center, www.holisticmed.com/aspartame

Fiber Helps Control Diabetes

PGX is in a product I use as a base for smoothies. This powder also
has whey for protein which is important especially as you age. It is also
something we sell in our shop. I add extra organic whey and fruit. It is
in several flavors. It is also in capsules but I think in this form it is a bit
pricey. PGX is "Konjac" a fiber substance and some other types of
fiber. Fiber offers many health benefits. Another good blend is apple
fibre, apple pectin and guar gum.

Novel fibers may blunt blood sugar spikes

By Nathan Gray, 08-Oct-2010

Related topics: Fibres and carbohydrates, Diabetes

Formulating foods with a novel functional fiber may reduce blood
sugar spikes after eating, according to a new study.

The research paper, published European Journal of Clinical Nutrition,
suggests that as little as 7.5 grams of PGX – a novel fiber supplement –
can reduce blood glucose responses over a two hour period by 50
percent, and can reduce post prandial responses by up to 28 percent.

The researchers, led by Prof. Jennie Brand-Miller from the University
of Sydney, stated that PGX has "biologically important, dose-related
effects on acute and delayed (second meal) postprandial glycemia."

The study was performed in partnership with researchers from Factors Group R & D, and InovoBiologic Inc. The study was also supported by InovoBiologic Inc, who also supplied the study with PGX.

Fabulous fiber

There is increasing evidence from long term studies to suggest that diets containing high quantities of whole grains and dietary fiber are associated with reduced risk of type 2 diabetes.

Controlled trials, have found that higher intake of cereal fiber leads to improvements in insulin sensitivity, whereas soluble fiber reduces postprandial glycemia, as well as serum lipids.

But despite awareness of the health benefits associated with dietary fiber, intakes have remained at about half the recommended level of 14 g per 1000 kcal.

Researchers noted supplementation of the diet with purified 'functional' dietary fibers "may be an option to increase fiber intake."

"Although both insoluble and soluble fibers can be used this way, soluble fibers that develop viscosity in solution appear to provide greater benefits for metabolism," added the authors.

Previous research has mainly focused on the ability of fiber preparations to improve lipid metabolism, however reductions in postprandial glycemia (often known as glycemic 'spikes') have increasingly been seen as an important part of the management and prevention of pre-diabetic glucose

intolerance and type-2 diabetes.

PolyGlycopleX (PGX) is a newly developed highly viscous polysaccharide complex that is reported to demonstrate a delayed onset of peak viscosity, "allowing for a more palatable and easy-to-use functional fiber,"state the authors.

The new study investigated the effectiveness of two different forms of PGX (granules or capsules), in reducing postprandial glycemia.

Reduced responses

Results from the study showed that the highest dose of the granular PGX (7.5 grams) dissolved in water and consumed with a carbohydrate meal at breakfast time, reduced the blood glucose responses by 50 percent.

The effectiveness of PGX granules was also related to timing, with researchers observing consumption within 15 minutes of the start of the meal reduced glycemia as effectively as when taken with the meal (up to 28 percent improvement) – however such effects were not found when taken at 45 or 60 minutes before the meal.

In contrast, PGX consumed as capsules did not produce immediate lowering of glycemia, but had important 'second meal' effects – improving glucose tolerance at breakfast time by up to 28 percent when consumed with the previous evening meal.

Beneficial effects

"These findings indicate that the effectiveness of PGX is dependent on dose, timing of consumption and physical form," stated the researchers.

They stated that the precise timing of ingestion for the PGX was not critical, because consumption between 15 minutes before and after the start of the meal was seen to be effective.

The authors noted that the beneficial effects of functional fibers are highly dependent on the food matrix, adding that unpublished data has suggested PGX to be "just as effective when sprinkled on food as dissolved in water."

They stated that further research was needed "to evaluate the long-term health benefits of this promising viscous polysaccharide."

Source: European Journal of Clinical Nutrition

Published online ahead of print, doi: 10.1038/ejcn.2010.199

"Effects of PGX, a novel functional fibre, on acute and delayed postprandial glycaemia"

Authors: J.C. Brand-Miller, F.S. Atkinson, R.J. Gahler, V. Kacinik, M.R. Lyon, S. Wood

Probiotic information - http://www.usprobiotics.org/basics.asp

Helps digestion, fights infection, helps diabetes with enzymes too.

Why I Advise Against Margarine

This is from my blog http://naturalhealthnews.blogspot.com/2010/09/margarine-not-hearthealthy.html

From my web site http://www.leaflady.org/fatfacts1.htm

Make your own garlic oil: see below article. This is also good for ear aches and can help avoid antibiotic use in this instance.

Garlic Oil Appears to Reverse Diabetes-Linked Heart Disease

New research with rats shows that supplementation with garlic oil may improve problems in heart function that are related to diabetes.

The study, published in the Journal of Agricultural and Food Chemistry, suggests that cardiac abnormalities induced by diabetes can be reversed in as little as 16 days of garlic oil supplementation.

"Our results show that garlic oil supplementation for diabetic rats leads to several alterations at multiple levels in hearts including cardiac contractile functions and structures, myosin chain gene expressions, oxidative stress and apoptosis and related signaling activities," wrote the researchers, led by Wei-Wen Kuo from the China Medical University in Taiwan.

Diabetes mellitus is a major risk factor in the development of cardiovascular disease, accounting for 80% of all diabetic mortality. Damage to cardiac function is well documented in diabetes, and death from heart disease is known to be between two and four times higher in patients with diabetes than in those without diabetes.

Garlic has been suggested to exhibit several health benefits, including inhibiting enzymes involved in lipid synthesis, decreasing platelet aggregation, preventing lipid peroxidation and increasing antioxidant status.

Previous studies have suggested that garlic oil could protect the cardiovascular system. However, the mechanism by which garlic oil protects diabetes-induced cardiomyopathy is unclear. The new study investigated the effect of garlic oil on the cardiac function of rats induced with diabetes.

Diabetes-related cardiac dysfunctions were dose-dependently relieved through administration of garlic oil. The researchers observed diabetes to significantly decrease heart rate, which was dose dependently reversed to control levels by garlic oil feeding.

Garlic oil was also reported to reverse the effects of diabetes on cardiac output and the heart's pumping capacity in a dose-dependent manner. Diabetic rats also showed significantly decreased levels of myosin heavy chains—key contractile proteins in the heart—which were dose-dependently attenuated by garlic oil.

The researchers concluded that "garlic oil possesses significant potential for protecting hearts from diabetes-induced cardiomyopathy." They added that garlic oil reduces oxidative stress and counteracts activations of up-regulated cell suicide signals, and as such could be considered to possess potential in protecting hearts from diabetic cardiomyopathy.

They added that further studies were needed, "to investigate the individual garlic oil constituent compounds on improving diabetic cardiac dysfunction."

Journal of Agricultural and Food Chemistry Published online ahead of print.

MAKE YOUR OWN GARLIC OIL

Organic garlic is best. Extra virgin olive oil cold press, not sold in plastic bottles To make garlic oil, which can be used in small amounts on salads or saved for medicinal purposes, blend one cup of chopped, peeled garlic cloves and cover with olive oil in a labeled jar, and then cap tightly. Keep in a cupboard and let the garlic be absorbed into the oil for a week, but shake the jar several times a day.

After 7 days strain out the garlic, and keep the liquid in the refrigerator. Warm at room temp before using as ear drop.

Save garlic and eat a teaspoon or so daily, or add to food.

Use this oil externally on wounds for adults, internally, or in salads, especially when swift cleansing action and antibacterial action is needed. A few drops of the oil can often help with low grade body infections and ear ache.

Turn Your Herbal Oils into a Salve

To turn your oil into a salve add 1 to 1 ½ ounces of melted beeswax into the herbal oil mix, keeping the temperature of the oil and the beeswax as close to the same temperature as you can. Stir constantly as it thickens and cools.

Pour into sterilized glass wide mouth jars, put on lid and store in the refrigerator. Salve should keep in the refrigerator for up to a year.

See also - http://www.herballegacy.com/Earaches.html

Hypoglycemia - Garlic also enhances the production of insulin and helps lower blood sugar levels. Experiments in India were reported in Lancet, the British medical journal. There is some indication that onions and garlic have a positive effect in diabetes.

...Just go for that onion sandwich ;)

Neuropathy: Cayenne- Capsaicin is an active ingredient in cayenne. Cayenne salve can be used topically to reduce pain and also help improve capillary circulation. Using cayenne extract or a capsule at meal time helps also. Cayenne can help stimulate pancreatic and digestive enzymes.

Garlic helps reduce triglycerides and this is much better to keep under 150 that to worry about cholesterol. Cholesterol lowering drugs can cause neuropathy.

Vitamin E

According to research by biochemist Dr. Ray Peat, persons with diabetes should take 1600 to 2000 IU vitamin E daily to off-set the ravages of diabetic retinopathy and circulatory restriction leading to loss of toes, et al. http://www.leaflady.org/Diabetic_Health.htm

To do this you should use non soy based vita E and start at 100 IU dail working up slowly to the suggested level. This is especially true if taking any blood thinning drugs or for people with hypertension. It is a well proven suggestion by science. Dr Peat is a biochemist with a PhD.

"Thus, vitamin E may potentially provide additional risk reduction for the development of retinopathy or nephropathy in addition to those achievable through intensive insulin therapy alone. Vitamin E is a low-cost, readily available compound associated with few known side effects; thus, its use could have a DRAMATIC socioeconomic impact if found to be efficacious in delaying the onset of diabetic retinopathy and/or nephropathy." (emphasis added) From Diabetes Care 22:1245-1251 1999

This was a crossover study on 36 patients who have Type I diabetes for less than 10 years. The dose evaluated was 1800 I.U. per day. Before taking vitamin E, retinal blood flows in these subjects was significantly lower than in the non-diabetic population. Both retinal blood flow and creatinine clearance were significantly normalized when subjects received vitamin E. The patients with the worst reading improved the most. The vitamin had no effect on blood glucose levels, and therefore would not interfere with insulin therapy.

(The following is from Stichting Orthomoleculaire Educatie (Orthomolecular Education Foundation) Antwerpsestraat 1a, 2587 AE Den Haag, The Netherlands. Their English language website is http://www.soe.nl/home.htm)

A poor vitamin-E status (lipid standardized plasma-vitamin E below the median) was associated with an almost quadruple risk of NIDDM (relative risk 3.9). The strong protective influence of vitamin E, as shown in these findings, supports the hypothesis that free-radical damage is a causal factor in the development of NIDDM.

(Increased risk of non-insulin dependent diabetes mellitus at low plasma vitamin E concentrations: a four year follow up study in men. (Salonen JT et al (1995); BMJ, 311:1124-1127, Oct. 28)

Vinegar Helps Keep Your Blood Sugar in Balance

Put Vinegar in Everything

(start with 1 tsp in a glass of water 15-20 minutes before meals - work up to 1 tablespoon, start once a day and work up to 3x a day. Use Raw apple cider vinegar - Bragg is a good . Helps many other things...AND just avoid white bread...There is more about vinegar on my web site at leaflady.org)

Vinegar does not confront Alzheimer's directly but there is evidence that vinegar sinks risk factors that may lead to memory decline and dementia -- namely, high blood sugar, insulin resistance, diabetes and prediabetes, and weight gain. Studies at Arizona State University have found that vinegar can curb appetite and food intake, helping prevent weight gain and obesity. Swedish investigators agree.

In one study, downing two or three tablespoons of vinegar with white bread cut expected rises in insulin and blood sugar by about 25 percent. Pour on the vinegar -- add it to salad dressings, eat it by the spoonful, even mix it into a glass of drinking water.

Vitamin Therapy for Diabetes

Diabetes: Dr. Klenner noted back in 1951 that the urine in his patients showed a reducing substance; severe virus infections will allow sugar to spill into the urine. Vitamin C acts as a reducing agent and it would appear that diabetes has been induced.

He reported the story of a seven year old diabetic, who developed measles, and his insulin requirements went from 5 units to more than 90 units a day, but with one gram of Vitamin C every four hours his infection and elevated blood sugar came under control. In these diabetic cases, the Vitamin C can be cut back to reasonable levels after the infection is under control. Large prolonged doses of "Vitamin C might prove undesirable due to its dehydrating and diuretic powers."

He feels that the pathological condition in this case means that adrenaline was flooding the boy's system. The regulator of the adrenaline mechanism had been removed so the constant supply caused a prolonged vascular constriction. This action on the blood vessels creates asphyxia of the tissues leading to acidosis. This acidity leads to adrenaline hyperglycemia. "Slight blood sugar elevation can be controlled with sodium bicarbonate. This vascular constriction is operative in the pancreas and could restrict the production of insulin and pancreatic enzymes."

As a matter of fact Dr. Klenner had been studying the effects of ten grams of C per day orally in patients with diabetes mellitus; 60% were able to control the condition with diet and C. The other 40% were able to reduce the insulin dose. Wounds healed more readily. The C assists the liver in its function of carbohydrate metabolism.

Generally we suggest 10 GRAMS daily of vitamin C for people with diabetes

It may not be news that a healthy diet plays a role in keeping type 2 diabetes at bay, but exactly which dietary components are most important is less well understood. A 2008 study sheds light on this question, suggesting that eating more fruit and vegetables rich in vitamin C is one way to reduce diabetes risk.

Make vitamin C a priority

These findings come out of the European Prospective Investigation of Cancer–Norfolk (EPIC–Norfolk) study, a long-term research effort focused on determining how nutrition and lifestyle factors affect risk of chronic diseases such as cancer, diabetes, and heart disease.

To arrive at the latest results, researchers collected diet information and blood samples from 21,831 men and women aged 40 to 75 years, who lived in Norfolk, England, and were free of diabetes at study enrollment. Researchers tracked new cases of diabetes in the group during 12 years of follow-up.

Study participants with the highest blood levels of vitamin C were 62% less likely to develop diabetes than those with the lowest vitamin C levels. Men and women who ate the most fruit and vegetables were 22% less likely to develop diabetes than those who ate the least. When considering fruit separately, the researchers found that people consuming the most fruit were 30% less likely to develop diabetes than those consuming the least.

The finding that vitamin C levels are more strongly correlated with reduced diabetes risk than fruit and vegetable intake may lead you to conclude that a supplement is the answer, but avoid this trap: The study authors note that errors are common when measuring what people eat and approximately 90% of the vitamin C intake in the study group came from fruit and vegetables, not dietary supplements.

The study authors conclude that the results, "re-endorse the public health message of the beneficial effect of increasing total fruit and vegetable intake."

Getting the C you need from food

Vitamin C is important for reducing diabetes risk, but where you get this superstar nutrient is even more critical. Use the following tips to "C" your way to better health.

• Start your day with fruit. Add frozen fruit to your oatmeal. The hot cereal will thaw the fruit and you'll get a dose of vitamin C.

• Try frozen and fresh. Fresh fruit is terrific when in season, but don't shy away from frozen. A half cup of frozen peaches provides more than 100% of daily C and a half cup of strawberries provides more than 50%.

• Enjoy citrus. Try oranges, tangerines, and even lemons. A squeeze of lemon juice into your tea or water is an easy way to add C into your diet.

• Don't skip veggies. Many focus on fruit for vitamin C, but red, yellow, and green peppers; broccoli; Brussels sprouts; and even kohlrabi contain ample C.

• Avoid boiling veggies. This can remove vitamin C; instead, steam, sauté, and stir-fry.

• Go tropical. Papayas, mangos, and pineapple all are excellent sources of vitamin C.

(Arch Intern Med 2008;168:1493–9)

Another Nutrition Resource

My main concern about Dr Lam is that he suggests canola oil which is known to be a negative oil for health and a trans fat, as well as GMO but he has good information otherwise.

http://www.drlam.com/articles/Diabetes.asp#Diabetes%20Protocol

Vitamin B1 Lowers Blood Sugar

The fact is that your body requires balanced blood sugar levels to stay healthy—to fight fat, to maintain optimal cholesterol levels and to ensure healthy inflammatory responses. Unfortunately, even a few weeks' worth of over eating, holiday stress, sleepless nights and lots of sugary snacks are capable of setting off a vicious cycle of metabolic mayhem that can be hard to get back under control.

The good news, however, is that with a little extra help, you can resume the maintenance of healthy blood sugar levels—and according to a new study, a daily dose of a single B vitamin, thiamine, may be the key to your success.

As part of this randomized, double-blind, placebo-controlled clinical trial, 24 subjects with blood sugar imbalances were given either 150 mg of thiamine (also known as vitamin B1) or a placebo for one month. None of the subjects had received any pharmacological intervention prior to the study period.

Blood tests were used to evaluate each subject for key metabolic factors both before and after the 30-day trial—with a focus on fasting blood glucose, hemoglobin A1C (a long-term measure of blood sugar control), creatinine (a marker of kidney function), lipid levels (including HDL cholesterol, LDL cholesterol and triglyceride levels) plus inflammatory markers (including C-reactive protein, IL-6, and TNF-alpha) and levels of both leptin and adiponectin, two hormones that play a critical role in glucose control and fat metabolism.

Results at the end of the 30-day trial showed that thiamine supplementation helped to maintain both healthy glucose and leptin levels1—which means that one 150 mg dose of this critical B vitamin per day in conjunction with your healthy lifestyle and diet may offer all the extra support you need to keep your blood sugar levels healthy this New Year. This optimal dose of thiamine is available to you now as the fat-soluble form of vitamin B1, called Benfotiamine, from Vitamin Research Products.

Reference:

1. González-Ortiz M, Martínez-Abundis E, Robles-Cervantes JA, Ramírez-Ramírez V, Ramos-Zavala MG.

Effect of thiamine administration on metabolic profile, cytokines and inflammatory markers in drug naïve patients with type 2 diabetes. Eur J Nutr. 2010 Jul 23. Published Online Ahead of Print." from VRP

Snack Lowers Blood Sugar

Eating a small, high-protein, low-carbohydrate snack two hours before breakfast resulted in lower blood glucose levels for participants with type 2 diabetes in a recent study. High post-meal blood glucose levels puts people with diabetes at risk for cardiovascular disease, a leading cause of death.

Because previous research shows that people who eat breakfast have lower blood glucose levels after the second meal of the day, researchers at Newcastle University conducted a small study to see if a small snack before breakfast would have a similar ameliorating effect on blood glucose levels after breakfast. Ten men and women with type 2 diabetes compared their blood glucose levels after just eating breakfast one day, with their blood glucose levels when eating a snack of 30 grams of soya beans and 75 grams of yogurt two hours before eating breakfast the next day. Blood glucose levels were nearly 40 percent lower on the day the participants ate the pre-breakfast snack. Although the researchers plan to conduct more research into the best timing and composition of the pre-breakfast snack, they suggest that this study "can be applied simply and practically to improve post-breakfast hyperglycemia in people with type 2 diabetes."

http://www.diabetesselfmanagement.com/Blog/Diane-Fennell/snack-drastically-reduces-post-mealglucose-in-study/

Magnesium

Basically magnesium (Mg) makes insulin work more effectively, one reason my energy formula ADVENTURx helps people with diabetes. Low magnesium (Mg) levels may increase the risk of complications in type 2 diabetics A new study from a team of Brazilian researchers has found that low levels of magnesium may worsen the symptoms of type 2 diabetes, as this often results in low levels of insulin and elevated blood sugar.

The researchers reported their findings in the journal Clinical Nutrition. They said that a diabetic's ability to control blood sugar levels is closely tied to their magnesium levels, as the mineral plays an important role in insulin receptor cells.

The findings are the second in a string of research connecting magnesium to healthy insulin levels. In fact, a study published in the latest issue of the journal Diabetes, Obesity and Metabolism found that taking oral magnesium supplements may help individuals who have become insulin resistant avoid developing type 2 diabetes.

For the current study, researchers from the University of Sao Paulo measured the blood sugar and magnesium levels of 51 patients who were being treated for type 2 diabetes. They found that 77 percent of the participants were magnesium deficient. Furthermore, the lower an individual's magnesium levels, the higher their blood sugar levels were.

The researchers said that combination of chronically high blood sugar levels and low magnesium may increase the risk of major diabetes complications, including kidney disease. They recommended that doctors test their diabetic patients for magnesium levels and provide appropriate treatment based on the results.

"Analysis of magnesium status in the routine assessment of such patients, or at least for those who are not able to reach the desired glycemic standards, would be useful in evaluating the risks relating to chronic complications in diabetes," the researchers wrote in their report. "Such strategy may help the management of type 2 diabetes and reduce the risk of long-term severe complications."

Something I've been saying for years, supported by another health writer.

The vinegar drink from Bragg helps with this too. http://www.leaflady.org/healing_with_vinegar.htm

I have tested ionic magnesium and I am seeing this benefit even though I am not a person with diabetes.

http://www.mineralifeonline.com/default.cfm?RID=1156&TID=2

Magnesium is necessary for both the action of insulin and the manufacture of insulin.

Magnesium is a basic building block to life and is present in ionic form throughout the full landscape of human physiology. Without insulin though, magnesium doesn't get transported from our blood into our cells where it is most needed. When Dr. Jerry Nadler of the Gonda Diabetes Center at the City of Hope Medical Center in Duarte, California and his colleagues placed 16 healthy people on magnesium-deficient diets, their insulin became less effective at getting sugar from their blood into their cells where it's burned or stored as fuel. In other words, they became less insulin sensitive, or what is called insulin resistant. And that's the first step on the road to both diabetes and heart disease.

A new study published in the journal Clinical Nutrition from a team of Brazilian researchers has found that low levels of magnesium worsens the symptoms of type 2 diabetes, as this often results in low levels of insulin and elevated blood sugar. The research indicates that a diabetic's ability to control blood sugar levels is closely tied to their magnesium levels, as the mineral plays an important role in insulin receptor cells. Another study published in the journal Diabetes, Obesity and Metabolism found that taking oral magnesium supplements helps individuals who have become insulin resistant avoid developing type 2 diabetes. These are just the latest in a long string of studies that the medical establishment and mainstream diabetes organizations continue to ignore. We know this because they continue to refuse to prescribe magnesium supplementation or treatments that can make all the difference in a diabetic's life.

Diabetes mellitus is positively associated with magnesium depletion, which in turn contributes to metabolic complications of diabetes including vascular disease and osteoporosis. Intracellular depletion is directly connected to the impaired ability of insulin to increase intracellular magnesium during insulin deficiency or insulin resistance.

Insulin is a common denominator, a central figure in life, as is magnesium. The task of insulin is to store excess nutritional resources. This system is an evolutionary development used to save energy and other nutritional necessities in times (or hours) of abundance in order to survive in times of hunger. Little do we appreciate that insulin is not just responsible for regulating sugar entry into the cells but also magnesium, one of the most important substances for life. It is interesting to note here that the kidneys are working at the opposite end, physiologically dumping from the blood excess nutrients that the body does not need or cannot process in the moment.

Controlling the level of blood sugars is only one of the many functions of insulin.

Insulin plays a central role in storing magnesium but if our cells become resistant to insulin, or if we do not produce enough insulin, then we have a difficult time storing magnesium in the cells where it belongs. When insulin processing becomes problematic, magnesium gets excreted through urine instead, and this is the basis of what is called magnesium-wasting disease.

There is a strong relationship between magnesium and insulin action.

Magnesium is important for the effectiveness of insulin. A reduction of magnesium in the cells strengthens insulin resistance.[1],[2]

Low serum and intracellular magnesium concentrations are associated with insulin resistance, impaired glucose tolerance, and decreased insulin secretion.[3],[4],[5] Magnesium improves insulin sensitivity thus lowering insulin resistance. Magnesium and insulin need each other. Without magnesium, the pancreas won't secrete enough insulin—or the insulin it secretes won't be efficient enough—to control our blood sugar.

Magnesium in our cells helps the muscles to relax, but if we can't store magnesium because the cells are resistant then we lose it. Losing magnesium makes the blood vessels constrict, affecting our energy levels and causing an increase in blood pressure. We begin to understand the intimate connection between diabetes and heart disease when we look at the closed loop between declining magnesium levels and declining insulin efficiency.

Though it would be a long stretch to compare insulin with chlorophyll, we are walking a trail at the very nuclear core of life. It's the magnesium trail and we find to our surprise that it takes us into intimate contact with the very structure and foundation of life. The dedication of this chapter is to the beauty of magnesium, to its meaning in life, in health, and in medicine.

Every part of life is in love with magnesium—except allopathic medicine, which just cannot accept it in all its light, flame and beauty.

Thousands of years ago the Chinese named it the beautiful metal and they were seeing something pharmaceutical medicine does not want to see for there is little money to be made from something so common.

In a study from Taiwan, the risk of dying from diabetes was inversely proportional to the level of magnesium in the drinking water.[6]

Dr. Jerry L. Nadler

Insulin resistance and magnesium depletion result in a vicious cycle of worsening insulin resistance and decrease in intracellular $Mg(2+)$ which limits the role of magnesium in vital cellular processes.[7] Magnesium is an important cofactor for enzymes involved in carbohydrate metabolism, so anything threatening magnesium levels threatens overall metabolism.

Large epidemiologic studies in adults indicate that lower dietary magnesium and lower serum magnesium are associated with increased risk for type 2 diabetes.[8],[9]

Redistribution of magnesium into cells may cause lower magnesium levels in the serum. Insulin causes this effect.

Researchers at the Institute of Internal Medicine, University of Palermo wrote, "Intracellular magnesium concentration has also been shown to be effective in modulating insulin action (mainly oxidative glucose metabolism), offset calcium-related excitation-contraction coupling, and decrease smooth cell responsiveness to depolarizing stimuli. A poor intracellular magnesium concentration, as found in noninsulin-dependent diabetes mellitus (NIDDM) and in hypertensive patients, may result in a defective tyrosine-kinase activity at the insulin receptor level and exaggerated intracellular calcium concentration."[10]

The link between diabetes mellitus and magnesium deficiency is well known. A growing body of evidence suggests that magnesium plays a pivotal role in reducing cardiovascular risks and may be involved in the pathogenesis of diabetes itself.

Dr. Jerry L. Nadler

Magnesium improves and helps correct insulin sensitivity, which is the fundamental defect that characterizes pre-diabetes, metabolic syndrome and even full-blown diabetes and heart disease.

An intracellular enzyme called tyrosine kinase requires magnesium to allow insulin to exert its blood sugar-lowering effects. In several studies, daily oral magnesium supplementation substantially improved insulin sensitivity by 10 percent and reduced blood sugar by 37 percent. [11],[12]

Magnesium also helps correct abnormal lipoprotein patterns. We would expect to find larger improvements in this increased insulin sensitivity if magnesium is supplemented in a correct way, meaning through transdermal and oral methods combined with using liquid magnesium chloride (magnesium oil) as compared to the very inefficient oral solid forms commonly used.

Improved insulin sensitivity from magnesium replacement can markedly reduce triglyceride levels.

[13] Reduced triglyceride availability, in turn, reduces triglyceride-rich particles, such as very-low density lipoprotein (VLDL) and small low-density lipoprotein (small LDL), both of which are powerful contributors to heart disease. Magnesium supplementation can also raise levels of beneficial high density lipoprotein (HDL).[14]

Insulin regulates intracellular magnesium levels via activation of Na+/Mg2+ exchange. Insulin's effect on Na/Mg exchange may explain the low cellular magnesium levels observed in vivo under hyperinsulinemic conditions.[15]

Magnesium and insulin need each other. Without magnesium, our pancreas won't secrete enough insulin—or the insulin it secretes won't be efficient enough—to control our blood sugar. Insulin is a hormone, and like many hormones, insulin is a protein. Insulin is secreted by groups of cells within the pancreas called islet cells. Insulin has many more functions than we realize. It regulates the following:

• Lifespan—Lower insulin levels equate to a longer life.

• Blood sugar

• Blood lipids

• Excess nutrients (from glucose, carbs and calories) and converts them to fat

• Muscle building

• Protein storage

• Magnesium levels in our body

• Calcium levels in the body

• Retains sodium levels

• Cell division

• Growth hormone

• Liver functions

• Sex hormones, estrogen, progesterone, testosterone

• Cholesterol in the body

• Fat in our body

Magnesium is a cofactor for multiple enzymes involved in carbohydrate metabolism.[16] Adipocyte cells placed in low-magnesium media show reduction in insulin-stimulated glucose uptake.

[17]Magnesium deficiency is associated with increased intracellular calcium levels, which may lead to insulin resistance. Low erythrocyte magnesium content increases membrane micro viscosity, which may

impair insulin interaction with its receptor.[18] Tyrosine kinase activity is decreased in muscle insulin receptors of rats fed a low-magnesium diet.[19] These findings indicate that magnesium deficiency directly affects insulin signaling.

When magnesium levels fall, hyper secretion of adrenalin and insulin compensate. Their increased secretions help maintain the constancy of the levels in intracellular magnesium in the soft tissues.

Plasma and intracellular magnesium concentrations are tightly regulated by insulin. But Dr. Ron Rosedale says that, "Extra insulin floating around in the blood causes plaque build-up. They didn't know why, but we know that insulin causes endothelial proliferation. Every step of the way, insulin is causing cardiovascular disease. It fills the body with plaque, it constricts the arteries, it stimulates the sympathetic nervous system, and it increases platelet adhesiveness and coagulability of the blood."

So as we can see, when magnesium levels drop there is a cascade of physiological problems that corrupt the heart of our health.

Statin Drugs Linked to Higher Risk of Diabetes

http://content.onlinejacc.org/cgi/content/abstract/57/14/1535

So why do they want you to take this?????

Red Yeast Rice is a statin also.

More of what many doctors and I have been saying for years: Statins are just a way to make $$$ for Big PhRMA and the patents are running out. Statin drugs are not good for your health.

Trans fats boost risk of sudden cardiac death

Trans fats, found in hydrogenated vegetable oils and some types of interesterified fats, both of which are used in many processed foods, elevate blood sugar, promote weight gain, and increase the risk of heart attack. In a study of more than 86,000 nurses over 26 years, Harvard University researchers found that consumption of trans fats was strongly related to sudden cardiac death – literally dropping dead – among women with preexisting heart disease.

Women who consumed the most trans fats had more than three times the risk of sudden cardiac death.

Chiuve SE. American Heart Journal, 2009;158:761-767.

Cinnamon - New study by Richard Anderson at the U.S. Department of Agriculture has found that cinnamon may help reduce risk factors that are associated with both heart disease and diabetes.

For this study, 22 obese subjects were recruited, all of whom had what's called "impaired blood glucose values," which means their blood sugar wasn't well controlled and they were at a higher risk for diabetes.

When blood sugar levels are too high, the body produces an abundance of insulin, also known as the "fat-storage hormone" or "the hunger hormone." The cells become resistant to this excess insulin, basically ignoring it while it "knocks" on the cell doors so it can get in to dump that extra sugar. You wind up with high blood sugar and high insulin, a condition known as insulin resistance.

While it's possible to have this kind of condition and not be overweight, it's pretty rare. According to the National Diabetes Information Clearinghouse, most people with insulin resistance develop full blown Type 2 diabetes within 10 years unless they lose 5 to 7 percent of their body weight. People with this condition are also much more at risk for developing cardiovascular disease.

In the present study, the volunteers were randomly divided into two groups. One group got a placebo while the other got 250 mg of water-soluble cinnamon extract, which they took twice a day in addition to their usual diet. The researchers collected blood after an overnight fast right at the beginning of the study, then again after six weeks and another time after 12 weeks.

They were looking for changes in either blood glucose (sugar), antioxidant levels or both.

The results? Those who took the cinnamon extract improved their antioxidant levels by between 13 and 23 percent.

That part's not surprising, as cinnamon contains a number of antioxidants. The surprising finding of the study was that this improvement in antioxidant status was accompanied by improvements in fasting blood sugar.

Earlier studies -- also by Anderson and his team -- showed that cinnamon was effective in reducing not only blood sugar but also triglycerides and total cholesterol in people with Type 2 diabetes. While weight loss is the most effective means to reduce your risk for diabetes, this small study suggests that adding cinnamon to your favorite healthy dishes could be much more than just a flavor boost.

Excellent Nutrition Site and Food Plan

It helps to correct biochemistry,
http://ifnh.org/lifestyle_diet_wholefood_nutrition.htm

OLIVE OIL, Just 1 Tablespoon a Day – OMEGA 3

Serum Omega-3 Fatty Acids are Significantly Decreased in Patients with Type 2 Diabetes and Non-Alcoholic Fatty Liver Disease

"[Serum omega-3 polyunsaturated fatty acid and insulin resistance in type 2 diabetes mellitus and nonalcoholic fatty liver disease]," Zhu QQ, Li D, et al, Zhonghua Nei Ke Za Zhi, 2010; 49(4): 305-8. (Address:

Department of Endocrinology and Metabolism, Shaoxing People's Hospital, Shaoxing, Zhejiang Province 312000, China. E-mail: sxzqq@126.com).

In a study involving 51 patients with type 2 diabetes and NAFLD (non-alcoholic fatty liver disease), 50 patients with type 2 diabetes, 45 patients with NAFLD, and 42 healthy controls, results indicate that supplementation with omega-3 polyunsaturated fatty acids (PUFAs) may exert a beneficial role in patients with type 2 diabetes and NAFLD. Patients with type 2 diabetes and NAFLD showed significantly lower levels of omega-3 PUFAs compared to patients with type 2 diabetes or NAFLD and controls. Additionally, serum omega-3 PUFAs concentrations were negatively correlated with HOMA-IR, total cholesterol, triglycerides, and LDL cholesterol. Thus, the authors of this study conclude, "Serum omega-3PUFA is significantly decreased in patients with type 2 diabetes mellitus and NAFLD. Serum omega-3PUFA is negatively correlated with insulin resistance. Omega-3PUFA plays a very important role in the development of diabetes mellitus and NAFLD."

Aspartame: aspartame is in children's medicine commonly given for ear infection and other medical issues to make it sweet. It is also in augmentin and some seizure meds (aspartame is also associated with causing seizure, as does Splenda)

The Miscellany News

http://www.miscellanynews.com/mobile/2.1577//mobile/2.1577

Opinions

Aspartame: the FDA's dirty little secret

By Laura Smyth, Guest Columnist

Wednesday, September 22, 2010

Take a look around: Aspartame is everywhere...why yes, even at Vassar. While it's well-known for being the artificial sweetener in Equal and NutraSweet, according to the Aspartame Information Center, it's also in 6,000 other products ranging from certain brands of pudding, jam, cereal, ketchup, soda, fat free yogurt, breath mints, to gum-as an avid gum fiend, I was disturbed to learn that aspartame is an ingredient in my favorite gum: Orbit Bubblemint. In our body-obsessed society, it makes sense that people gravitate towards products with the least calories. Aspartame has 90 percent fewer calories than regular sugar, and is much sweeter-clearly, an attractive premise.

So what's all the fuss? Aspartame has been in a constant cloud of controversy-both because of safety concerns and the seemingly questionable circumstances surrounding its approval by the Food and Drug Administration (FDA). First the Department of Justice went after Searle, the manufacturer of NutraSweet, which contains aspartame, for fraud in one of its aspartame studies, and, as Dr. Christine Lydon noted in an article, even the National Soft Drink Association had been against the approval of aspartame in soft drinks.

The FDA had routinely denied aspartame approval for over a decade, until 1981, when a newly appointed commissioner of the FDA, Dr. Arthur Hull Hayes, took office and ultimately overruled the decision. There was never enough evidence for an official investigation-but just two years after this approval deal he left the FDA after allegations of impropriety and went to work for a public relations firm whose chief client was Searle, company that had patented aspartame in the first place.

According to the World Wide Health Center, David Reitz, founder of DORWay, a group of anti-aspartame activists, Dr. Betty Martini, creator of the Mission Possible World Health International organization, and a direct report from the U.S. Department of Health and Human Services, among others, there are 92 established symptoms attributed to aspartame use.

The FDA report states that these symptoms range from headaches to hives to, yes, even changes in one's menstrual pattern. If you were to Google "aspartame side effects"-do it, if you're curious-you'd easily find an abundance of sources screaming that it can literally kill you, among other horrible things like render you blind, cause seizures or give you cancer. At this point in time there haven't even been enough substantive studies published on the most horrible side effects of consuming too much aspartame, but the consumption of this sweetener over time, like the over consumption of many other things, can lead to noticeable damage. Moderation is the key.

It's easy to see why people might bend the truth in order to keep aspartame on the market-it's a multibillion dollar industry in a faltering economy. But why would so many other people, who stand to gain nothing financially, invest themselves in a campaign against aspartame if there's really nothing wrong with it?

So, hey-here we are at Vassar. If you try hard enough, you just might be able to hide from the majority of events making national news. But what about those things that don't make the news, and furthermore, those which directly affect your health, which perhaps are even deliberately hiding from you? You (try) to find the time to work out consistently and consciously, and (genuinely attempt to) eat well, glancing at caloric information on packaging when available. Fat-free, nearly calorie free, SCORE? Just check the ingredients prior to prancing in glee.

Vassar can do everything possible to ensure that quality food is served at the All Campus Dining Center or sold at the Retreat, but that being said, it's ultimately up to the student as to how he or she eats. That's us. As the poet Gerald Massey said: "They must find it hard, those who have taken authority as truth, rather than truth as authority." Just because something's legal and in front of you doesn't mean you should put it on your mouth. Don't blindly trust the FDA. Don't eat aspartame.

Lisa Marconi

Thu Sep 23 2010 16:10

The vast majority of scientific research NOT FUNDED BY THE ASPARTAME INDUSTRY proves that this substance is a dangerous neurotoxin and excitotoxin that stimulates brain cells to death - yes, even if you do not have a reaction from drinking or eating it, aspartame and its breakdown products are stored and accumulate in the cells until you reach a tipping point. That tipping point may be diagnosed as multiple sclerosis or any other of a range of neurologic problems. Just because ingesting the substance does not appear to have any bad effect on you at the time does mean you are not being adversely affected by it. This poison will ruin your health. Here are two good films about one woman's reaction to aspartame and her return to health: Sweet Misery and Sweet Remedy. You can find them at http://www.sweetremedy.tv

Anonymous

Type 2 diabetes linked to air pollution

BOSTON, Oct. 4, 2010

(UPI) -- There is a strong, consistent correlation between adult diabetes -- type 2 diabetes – and particulate air pollution, U.S. epidemiologists suggest.

Study leaders John Pearson and John Brownstein of the Children's Hospital Boston Informatics Program analyzed county-by-county data on PM2.5 pollution -- fine particulates of 0.1-2.5 nanometers in size – from the U.S. Environmental Protection Agency covering every county in the contiguous United States for 2004 and 2005.

The researchers examined the data along with data from the Centers for Disease Control and Prevention and the U.S. Census to track the prevalence of adult diabetes. They factored in known diabetes risk factors such as obesity, exercise, geographic latitude, ethnicity and population density.

The study, published in the journal Diabetes Care, found a strong and consistent association between diabetes prevalence and PM2.5 concentrations. For every 10 micrograms per cubic meter increase in PM2.5 exposure, there was a 1 percent increase in diabetes prevalence, the researchers learned.

"We didn't have data on individual exposure, so we can't prove causality, and we can't know exactly the mechanism of these people's diabetes," Brownstein said in a statement. "But pollution came across as a significant predictor in all our models."

The correlation was seen even at exposure levels below the current EPA safety limit, the study revealed.

Diagnosis and Treatment of Vitamin B12 Deficiency

I think this dose is too low based on historical data but good info B12 should be 2400-2800 mcg daily. B vitamins are crucial for people with diabetes. I suggest NUTRITIONAL YEAST, start with 1 tsp daily and work up to 1-2 TBSP daily. This also has all the B vitamins, amino acids - excellent protein source – and some minerals for health.

There is a type of organic nutritional yeast made by Diamond V and you get it at the feed store. It also comes as non-organic which is less money but I favor the organic.

This yeast is sold in health food stores at a very high price under the name EpiCor. If you pooled together you can get a bag (50 pounds) and divide it up. It will help you stay well during the winter and all year too. http://www.diamondv.com/products-specific/ XPC

VITAMIN B12 DEFICIENCY, ANEMIA

Vitamin B12, Cobalamin, Holotranscobalamin "Diagnosis and treatment of vitamin B12 deficiency—an update," Hvas AM, Nexo E, et al, Haematologica, 2006; 91(11): 1506-12. (Address: Department of Clinical Biochemistry, Aarhus University Hospital, Skejby, Denmark. E-mail: am.hvas@dadlnet.dk).

In a review article summarizing data regarding the diagnosis and treatment of vitamin B12 deficiency, the authors conclude that a daily dose of 1 mg (1000 mcg) vitamin B12, or injections of vitamin B12 every 2-3 months, may effectively treat vitamin B12 deficiency.

In terms of diagnosis, the authors recommend that the following groups be particularly suspected and examined for vitamin B12 deficiency: 1) patients with anemia which is unexplained; 2) patients with neurological symptoms which are unexplained; 3) patients with intestinal diseases; and 4) the elderly.

In terms of clinical measurements, plasma cobalamin has been considered the primary tool to assess vitamin B12 deficiency, although plasma holotranscobalamin (biologically active cobalamin) has recently been suggested to be a superior tool. Measuring methymelanonic acid may also used, mainly in unsettled cases. In terms of treatment, it has been found that 1000 mcg (1 mg) vitamin B12 taken orally daily or injections of vitamin B12 every 2-3 months may effectively treat established vitamin B12 deficiency.

Individuals who are vegetarians/vegans obtain very little vitamin B12 in their diet. Supplementation with B12 should be advised.

Certain drugs (eg; Glucophage/Metformin) cause B12 depletion, requiring B12 supplementation.

Garlic for Health and Diabetes

I am a real fan of garlic for health. It offers many benefits. It is also a remedy you can make on your own. I you prefer products, I suggest garlicwise.com (please use Dr. Gayle Eversole for reference) or one other that I have sold for years. My web site, www.leaflady.org, has a lot of information about garlic.

In Persia one of the traditional foods is pickled garlic, or pickled garlic with baby beets, an excellent approach to health.

To make you own, get several large organic garlic heads. Peel the cloves and place the cloves in a glass jar, pack pretty full. Cover with high quality extra virgin olive oil that is sold in glass bottles (dark or green glass is best as is unfiltered olive oil). Tightly cap.

Shake well and place in cupboard. Shake daily for a week.

Daily eat a few cloves of garlic along with a tablespoon of the oil. You can replenish the oil as you eat the garlic.

You can also cover the cloves with raw, apple cider vinegar. If using vinegar you have to use a plastic lid because metal and vinegar do not mix.

Garlic oil may reverse diabetes linked heart disease

By Nathan Gray, 30-Sep-2010

Related topics: Antioxidants, carotenoids, Nutritional lipids and oils, Cardiovascular health, Diabetes Problems in heart function related to diabetes may be improved by supplementation with garlic oil, according to new research with rats.

The study, published in the Journal of Agricultural and Food Chemistry, suggests that cardiac abnormalities induced by diabetes can be reversed in as little sixteen days of garlic oil supplementation.

"Our results show that garlic oil supplementation for diabetic rats leads to several alterations at multiple levels in hearts including cardiac contractile functions and structures, myosin chain gene expressions, oxidative stress, and apoptosis and related signaling activities," wrote the researchers, led by Wei-Wen Kuo from the China Medical University in Taiwan.

Diabetic risk

Diabetes mellitus is a major risk factor in the development of cardiovascular disease, accounting for 80 percent of all diabetic mortality.

Damage to cardiac function is well documented in diabetes, and death from heart disease is known to be between two and four times higher in patients with diabetes than those without diabetes.

Garlic (Allium sativum) has been suggested to exhibit several health benefits, including inhibiting enzymes involved in lipid synthesis, decreasing platelet aggregation, preventing lipid peroxidation, and increasing antioxidant status.

Garlic oil is commonly used in cooking and folk remedies.

Previous studies have suggested that garlic oil could protect the cardiovascular system. However, the mechanism by which garlic oil protects diabetes-induced cardiomyopathy is unclear.

The new study investigated the effects of garlic oil on the cardiac function of rats induced with diabetes.

Dose-dependent reversal

Diabetes related cardiac dysfunctions were dose-dependently relieved through administration with garlic oil.

The researchers observed diabetes to significantly decrease heart rate– which was dose-dependently reversed to control levels by garlic oil feeding.

Garlic oil was also reported to reverse the effects of diabetes on cardiac output and the hearts pumping capacity in a dose dependant manner.

Diabetic rats also showed significantly decreased levels of myosin heavy chains– key contractile proteins in the heart – which were dose dependently attenuated by garlic oil.

Significant potential

The researchers concluded that "garlic oil possesses significant potential for protecting hearts from diabetes-induced cardiomyopathy."

Adding that garlic oil reduces oxidative stress and counteracts activations of up-regulated cell suicide signals, and as such could be considered to possess potential in protecting hearts from diabetic cardiomyopathy.

"All of these phenomena might be associated with the antioxidant potential of garlic oil, which is attributed to the presence of organosulfur compounds that modulate the cardiac antioxidant activity," said the authors.

They added that further studies were needed, "to investigate the individual garlic oil constituent compounds on improving diabetic cardiac dysfunction."

Source: Journal of Agricultural and Food Chemistry

Published online ahead of print: 10.1021/jf101606s

"Cardiac Contractile Dysfunction and Apoptosis in Streptozotocin-Induced Diabetic Rats Are Ameliorated by Garlic Oil Supplementation"

Authors: H.C Ou, B.S Tzang, M.H. Chang, C.T Liu, H.W. Liu, C.K Lii, D.T Bau, P.N Chau, E.W Kuo

Garlic goes under trial for diabetes management

26-Mar-2004

UK researchers are to test whether garlic could be used to counter diabetes, promising renewed

interest in one of the most well-established dietary supplement products.

The scientists at Manchester Metropolitan University believe liquid garlic could prevent the damage to the eyes, kidneys, blood vessels and skin of diabetes patients caused by high sugar levels in a process known as glycation.

"Garlic in its liquid form has proved a potent block on glycation in a series of in-vitro tests we have conducted,"said Dr Nessar Ahmed, molecular biologist at the university's department of biological sciences.

"We are trying to understand why sugars destroy the body from the inside and have a particular interest in natural products and their therapeutic benefits."

The researcher is one of many looking at whether a natural product can help prevent diabetes or play a role in the treatment of the disease. Diabetes increased by one third during the 1990s due to the prevalence of obesity and an ageing population. If nothing is done to slow the epidemic, more than 333 million people in the world could have the disease by 2025, according to the International Diabetes Federation.

Garlic is already one of the best-selling herbal dietary supplement products in the United States, and in some European markets such as Germany and the UK, where sales increased 13 per cent in 2002.

There are thought to be more than 2,200 credible scientific papers on all aspects of garlic, including its chemistry, pharmacology, and clinical applications.

"One of the other things that people with diabetes have is increased free radical activity which can also have a role in these complications," said Dr Ahmed.

Garlic's antioxidant properties - thought to fight free radicals - ave been widely studied. It may also lower cholesterol levels, often hig in diabetics.

Dr Ahmed's team will carry out a clinical trial on 70 patients with type 2 diabetes at a hospital in Saudi Arabia. The researcher recently discovered that the key ingredient in aged garlic extract, sallylcysteine, slowed the glycation process.

Other British scientists have recently found that a compound extracted from garlic is effective against even the most antibiotic-resistant strains of MRSA, the 'hospital superbug' that now kills thousands of patients in the UK each year.

TYPE 2 DIABETES - Cinnamon, HbA1c, Systolic Blood Pressure, Diastolic Blood Pressure

"Glycated haemoglobin and blood pressure-lowering effect of cinnamon in multi-ethnic Type 2 diabetic patients in the UK: a randomized, placebo-controlled, double-blind clinical trial," Akilen R, Robinson N, et al, Diabet Med, 2010; 27(10): 1159-67. (Address: Faculty of Health and Human Science,

Thames Valley University, London, UK and Department of Investigative Sciences, Faculty of Medicine, Imperial College London and Brent Community services (National Health Service), London, UK).

In a randomized, placebo-controlled study involving 58 men and women with type 2 diabetes, results indicate that supplementation with cinnamon may exert beneficial effects. The subjects were randomized to 2 g of cinnamon or placebo daily for a period of 12 weeks. At intervention end, significant decreases in HbA1c (-.36%), mean systolic and diastolic blood pressures (-3.4 mm Hg and -5 mm Hg, respectively), fasting plasma glucose, waist circumference and body mass index was observed in the cinnamon group, compared with the placebo group. Thus, the authors of this study conclude, "Intake of 2g of cinnamon for 12 weeks significantly reduces the HbA1c, SBP and DBP among poorly controlled type 2 diabetes patients. Cinnamon supplementation could be considered as an additional dietary supplement option to regulate blood glucose and blood pressure levels along with conventional medications to treat type 2 diabetes mellitus.

Vitamin D May Help Prevent Diabetes – As I have said for years (D3 and Zinc for Type 1)

Vitamin D also is important to raise the effectiveness of the immune system which would go a long way in preventing colds, flu, and pneumonias. This is not just an issue for children or Type 1. Vitamin D is very crucial for adults, especially those in northern states. It is an inexpensive way to improve health in many ways and especially for anyone on dialysis. (With Kidney problems usually D2 is used although it is about half as effective as vitamin D3)

Exciting research also indicates a possible therapeutic role for vitamin D in preventing diabetes.

Vitamin D supplementation may reduce susceptibility to type II diabetes by slowing the loss of insulin sensitivity in people who show early signs of the disease. Researchers studied 314 adults without diabetes and gave them either 700 IU of vitamin D and 500 mg of calcium daily or a placebo for three years.[73] Among subjects who had impaired (slightly elevated) fasting glucose levels at the study's onset, those taking the active supplement had a smaller rise in glucose levels over three years than did the controls, as well as a smaller increase in insulin resistance. The researchers concluded that for older adults with impaired glucose levels, supplementing with vitamin D and calcium may help avert metabolic syndrome and type II diabetes.

Type I (insulin dependent) diabetes is an autoimmune condition, in which the body's immune system attacks its own insulin-producing pancreatic beta cells. Low vitamin D levels are associated with the development of autoimmune conditions,[40,74,75] including type I diabetes,38 and scientists have proposed that vitamin D supplementation may help prevent the disease.76

A very large population-based study in Europe demonstrated the powerful effect of vitamin D supplementation in protecting children against the development of type I diabetes.77 Data from 820 diabetics and 2,335 non-diabetic controls showed that children who received vitamin D supplements in infancy reduced their risk of developing type I diabetes by approximately 33%. The researchers believe that activated vitamin D may protect growing children from autoimmune attack on insulin producing cells of the pancreas.

THYROID & DIABETES: This is a very good article - Thyroid hormone assists insulin in moving glucose from the blood into cells. When thyroid levels are low, more insulin is needed to maintain normal glucose.

More insulin means more fat cell hyperplasia, which shows up as increased fat deposition, especially around hips, thighs and abdomen (truncal obesity), all of which point to suboptimal thyroid levels. http://www.holisticprimarycare.net/topics/topics-h-n/healthy-aging/94-the-clinical-picture-ofhypothyroidism

ACTOS and Bladder Cancer

WASHINGTON September 17, 2010 -- The FDA is investigating a possible link between pioglitazone (Actos) and bladder cancer, and, as a result, both of the available thiazolidinediones – pioglitazone and rosiglitazone (Avandia) -- are undergoing safety reviews.

The FDA said it initiated the pioglitazone review after it received preliminary data from a 10-year epidemiological study sponsored by Takeda.

An interim analysis of data from the study, which includes more than 193,000 patients with type 2 diabetes, revealed no statistically significant increase in bladder cancer among pioglitazone users compared with nonusers (hazard ratio 1.2, 95% CI 0.9 to 1.5), but "the risk of bladder cancer increased with increasing dose and duration of [pioglitazone] use, reaching statistical significance after 24 months of exposure."

Moreover, "results from two, three-year controlled clinical studies of Actos (the PROactive study and a liver safety study) demonstrated a higher percentage of bladder cancer cases in patients receiving Actos versus comparators," the FDA wrote in its announcement of the safety review.

The findings from PROactive are included in the current pioglitazone label in the "Precautions – Carcinogenesis, Mutagenesis, Impairment of Fertility" section.

Robert Spanheimer, MD, Takeda's medical director for pioglitazone, told MedPage Today that the FDA announcement and the data from the epidemiological study need to be "interpreted in the context of being interim results from a 10-year study."

Moreover, he pointed out, the data did not reach statistical significance for the primary endpoint of increased risk of bladder cancer.

The "investigators did a post-hoc analysis (of these preliminary data) that showed duration [of treatment] had an effect on the association," Spanheimer noted, leaving unsaid the fact that results of a post-hoc analysis should be considered no more than hypothesis-generating.

When asked if he thought today's FDA announcement was justified based on the data, he said Takeda "is interested in safety, as is the FDA." He declined to offer comment on the appropriateness of the announcement.

Spanheimer made his comments in a phone interview that was monitored by a Takeda public relations spokesperson.

The FDA said the safety review should not impact clinical care and advised that physicians continue to prescribe pioglitazone according to approved marketing indications and label directions. Patients using pioglitazone should continue to take the drug unless they are told to stop by their physician.

Over the last few years, pioglitazone has enjoyed a reputation as the "safer" TZD because, unlike rosiglitazone, it has not been linked to excess risk of cardiovascular events -- even though both drugs carry warnings about increased risk of congestive heart failure.

Rosiglitazone has twice been the subject of special hearings, and the FDA is still digesting results of the latest round of hearings at which advisers again recommended that the drug stay on the market, but with even tougher boxed warnings.

Rosiglitazone has also been the subject of congressional hearings about the way in which its maker, GlaxoSmithKline, controlled findings from clinical trials, and more such hearings are expected.

Through more than two years of controversy, pioglitazone was, by comparison, racking up published data that burnished its reputation: for slowing atherosclerosis, for treating psoriasis, for providing cardiovascular safety, and even -- in a phase I study -- for treating Alzheimer's disease.

The flurry of data -- good, bad, and equivocal -- for both of the TZDs have at best created confusion for physicians treating patients with diabetes mellitus -- confusion that continued through this year's American Diabetes Association meeting at which Leo Green, MD, MPH, of the University of Michigan, in Ann Arbor, summed up the debate this way for MedPage Today: "The first question is not whether to switch someone from Avandia to Actos, but whether they should be on either one at all."

Review supports health benefits of Spirulina

By Mike Stones, 13-Sep-2010

Related topics: Antioxidants, carotenoids, Cancer risk reduction, Cardiovascular health, Immune system

The 'encouraging' health benefits of spirulina; a blue-green algae used in dietary supplements and functional foods for its antioxidant properties, should promote further research, says a new review.

The potential health benefits of spirulina, which include immune health, cardiovascular health, and potential anti-cancer effects, should also encourage dietary supplementation, according to the review published in the journal Nutra Foods,

Entitled Potential health benefits of spirulina microalgae; a review of the existing literature, the article was written by Bob Capelli, vice president sales and Marketing of Cyanotech which produces and sells spirulina and Gerald Cysewski, the company's chief scientific officer.

Immune-stimulating - After reviewing studies looking at the health benefits of products made from the blue-green algae, the authors concluded that: "Spirulina shows potent immune-stimulating effects (and) …. anti-viral activity against a variety of harmful viruses."

It also "…shows promise as a cancer preventative agent and in the treatment of tumors," and has "… far ranging cardiovascular benefits including improvement of blood lipid profiles, prevention of atherosclerosis, and control of hypertension."

In humans, spirulina produces an immuno-stimulating effect by enhancing the resistance to infections, the capacity of influencing hemopoieses (the process by which new blood cells are formed) and stimulating the production of antibodies and cytokines.

Spirulina's anti-viral properties were noted both in simple water extracts and dried bomass. The authors concluded that the algae's anti-viral properties are derived both from its polysaccharides as well as other components.

In terms of cancer prevention, the authors acknowledged a shortage of human clinical research. But in animal studies they highlighted a numerous studies showing spirulina's potential to prevent carcinogenesis and to shrink tumours.

By contrast, the cardiovascular benefits of spirulina are described in many papers, according to the review article. A review published in 2009 noted several reports suggesting that spirulina may have a

beneficial effect in the prevention of cardiovascular diseases. Decreases in blood pressure and plasma lipid concentrations, especially triacylglycerols and low density lipoprotein-cholesterol have been demonstrated as a result of oral consumption of spirulina.

Health benefits

Further research into the potential of spirulina and its constituent pigment C-phycocyanin in the four areas noted promise to unlock further health benefits, noted the authors.

The authors reviewed a series of published studies, most of which appeared in the past 10 years.

Many studies investigated benefits from pure Spirulina biomass, but some also focused on extracts of spirulina or isolated compounds from spirulina. These were mainly C-phycocyanin, the blue-green pigment found only in spirulina and other species of blue-green microalgae.

Research into the health benefits of this uni-cellular, blue-green microalgae began in the 1970s and has accelerated during the past 10 years.

Source: NutraFoods

Volume 9, Pages 16-26

"Potential health benefits of spirulina microalgae; a review of the existing literature"

Authors: B. Capelli, G. Cysewski

Copyright - Unless otherwise stated all contents of this web site are © 2000/2010 - Decision News Media

SAS - All Rights Reserved -

Yellow Pea flower to improve insulin resistance http://www-t.decisionnewsmedia.com/r/?

id=h18f57333,5cd211f,5cd285d&p1=fD4QEMYsyb%2FvMy1EkktyJQ%3D%3D

Some Food Tips to Help Lower Blood Sugar

Dill pickle can lower your blood sugar up 20-40% when eaten with a sandwich.

The pickle juice is similar to having fresh squeezed lemon juice in water - one-tablespoon of lemon juice dropped the blood-sugar impact of a meal by 30%

Apple cider vinegar in water lowers blood sugar up to 55%

Avocado is a healthy food and high in fiber.

Sunshine 'can help you live longer by cutting risk of heart disease and diabetes'

http://www.telegraph.co.uk/news/uknews/5340854/Sunshine-can-help-you-live-longer-by-cutting-riskof-heart-disease-and-diabetes.html

Sunscreen: Vitamins C and B1 help keep you sun-screened. Tomatoes also help prevent sunburn.

Vitamins C and B1 help prevent diabetes, and can help cure it too.

Diabetes and the Nervous System

Canadian scientists found proof that diabetes can be triggered by the body's nervous system. For most researchers/scientists/people, Type 1 diabetes has been thought to be related strictly to an autoimmune response. However, animal studies revealed that counteracting the effects of neurons in the pancreas produced remarkable changes overnight allowing the islets to begin producing insulin normally. Dr. Salter stated "Mice with diabetes suddenly didn't have diabetes anymore." The researchers also found a strong similarity between type 1 and type 2 diabetes which were thought to be entirely different. Recognition of the link between the nervous system and various disease processes may eventually lead to the treatment and elimination of many other neuropathic related diseases. www.Canada.com. Dec. 2006.

Comment: Through viewing HTMA studies we have always emphasized not only a neurological link in many disease processes such as diabetes, but also an endocrine link. This neuro-endocrine link is involved in most all diseases and HTMA studies can help in revealing the underlying metabolic and nutritional disturbances associated with many health conditions. Metabolic Manifestation of Disease, Sympathetic-Parasympathetic. TEI Newsletter Vol. 3, 3, 1989

Herbs to help your health

Capsaicin is the component of cayenne that I have used for a very long time in pain treatment and nerve healing.

This supports the rationale for other natural treatment I have used for Type 1 (Astragalus and antiinflammatory Marshmallow root).

A reason also to consider turmeric but the dose has to be high (if you would like my turmeric article let me know), and why MSM and other things like vitamin C and E work for neuropathy and other forms of inflammation.

http://www.canada.com/nationalpost/news/story.html?id=a042812e-492c-4f07-8245-8a598ab5d1bf&k=63970&p=2

see MS comment on page 1

Just wish herbal medicine would get some credit here!

It is a good thing to use cayenne capsules, 35,000 heat unit strength. It does all kinds of good things I hope this can be of help to at least one person, and then I am happy.

This is a Bulgarian herbal extract. In 2000 I had an exchange student who taught me about the Bulgarian herbs and translated all the books for me. Today I met this fellow via twitter who is from Canada but sells these herbs as he is now in Bulgaria. I have used these herbs and they are really very good. You notice that it is the pancreas and thyroid that gets impact, a truly wise formula.

Special Formula for the Normalization of Blood Sugar

Action: It normalizes the functions of the endocrine system especially the pancreas and the thyroid. It has a powerful bio stimulating action, normalizes the blood sugar and promotes the rapid healing of wounds.

Additional effects: It has a strong tonic effect on the whole body and improves regeneration, blood circulation, and the elasticity of blood vessels. It also dramatically improves metabolism, the functions of the kidneys, lungs, and the liver.

250 Ml. Plastic Bottle

Contraindications: Allergies to bee honey or any other ingredients.

Dosage: Morning and evening 1-2 teaspoons in water, juice or other liquid.

Contains: bee Honey, extracts of Rhodiola Rosea, Ginkgo Biloba, Lycium, Ginseng, Nettle seeds, Goat's Rue, Sweet Root, Melissa, Valerian Root, Walnut.

Dr Briffa has some really good articles about diabetes.

http://www.drbriffa.com/2010/07/27/diabetes-costs-out-of-control-and-why-this-is-no-surprise-givenstandard-dietary-advice-for-diabetics/

The Importance of Chromium –

Chromium piconicotinate is crucial for people with diabetes. It can also be found in organic nutritional yeast or GTF factor yeast.

Most suggest 200 mcg daily however those in the know say it is more like 200, 3 times a day.

Chromium is the master regulator of insulin and involved in protein, fat, and carbohydrate metabolism.

Chromium is necessary for glucose metabolism, neurotransmiters, insulin performance, thyroid function, and hormonal balance.

Deficiency symptoms often include: hypoglycemia, aortic cholesterol, peripheral neuropathy, hypo/hyper thyroid, excess body weight, depression and ateriosclerosis.

Inflammation -

Usually diabetes is considered an inflammatory state and also a state of accelerated aging.

One thing that is promoted is the use of non-saturated fat in the diet which is probably not good when you think that fish oil, coconut oil, olive oil and real unsalted butter promote health. Of course the key is to use all fat in moderation but be sure to ignore the non-fat diet craze because your brain and all hormones require healthy fat to function.

There is a lot of new information and old information re-circulating, must be a need.

Mechanism found for omega-3 fatty acids in insulin resistance and inflammation

An article published in the September 3, 2010 issue of the journal Cell reports the discovery of researchers at the University of California, San Diego School of Medicine of the mechanism used by omega-3 fatty acids in lowering insulin resistance and chronic inflammation.

Recent research revealed that five members of a family of molecules known as G protein-coupled receptors respond to free fatty acids. Using cell cultures, Jerrold Olefsky, MD and colleagues found that exposure to omega-3 fatty acids activates one of these cellular receptors. The receptor, known as GPR120, is located on macrophages in mature fat cells and, when activated, prevents the macrophages from causing inflammation.

The researchers compared the effects of diets supplemented with the omega-3 fatty acids EPA and DHA in mice bred to lack the GPR120 receptor and normal mice. Prior to receiving EPA and DHA, both groups of animals received high fat diets for 15 weeks to induce obesity and insulin resistance.

While the normal mice experienced enhanced insulin sensitivity and reduced inflammation after 5 weeks of omega-3 supplementation, mice lacking the receptor failed to benefit from the omega-3 fatty acids. The insulin-sensitizing ability of EPA and DHA was the same or greater than that found for the drug rosiglitazone in a separate group of normal obese mice.

"It's just an incredibly potent effect," enthused Dr Olefsky, who is a professor of medicine and associate dean of scientific affairs for the UC San Diego School of Medicine. "The omega-3 fatty acids switch on the receptor, killing the inflammatory response."

"Omega-3s are very potent activators of GPR120 on macrophages -- more potent than any other anti-inflammatory we've ever seen," he remarked, adding that activation of GPR120 by omega-3 blocks all inflammatory pathways.

"This is nature at work," he observed. "The receptor evolved to respond to a natural product – omega-3 fatty acids – so that the inflammatory process can be controlled. Our work shows how fish oils safely do this, and suggests a possible way to treating the serious problems of inflammation in obesity and in conditions like diabetes, cancer and cardiovascular disease through simple dietary supplementation."

Women's Health and Diabetes

I think this is worth considering because it speaks to overall nutritional deficiency and it is directly related to young girls and women who have or are taking birth control pills (BCP). BCP can promote obesity and diabetes, also severe nutritional deficiency

http://www.leaflady.org/bcpillnutrition.htm

http://www.leaflady.org/somethoughts.htm

Lonza's L-carnitine may reduce diabetes during pregnancy

By Stephen Daniells, 02-Sep-2010

Related topics: Diabetes, Maternal & infant health

Daily supplements of L-carnitine tartrate during pregnancy may decrease levels of free fatty acids linked to insulin resistance and gestational diabetes, says a new study.

Insulin resistance during pregnancy can lead to gestational diabetes, which affects about 5-10 per cent of pregnancies. According to the American Diabetes Association, about a third of women who suffered from gestational diabetes during pregnancy develop type-2 diabetes in the following years.

Blood levels of the vitamin-like substance L-carnitine are already significantly reduced by the 12th week of pregnancy, and are reduced further before birth.

According to findings published in the Journal for Obstetrics and Gynecology (Gynakologischgeburtshilfliche Rundschau), daily supplements with two grams of L-Carnitine in the form of Lonza's Carnipure tartrate during pregnancy may reduce levels of free fatty acids in the blood, high levels of which are thought to be the main cause of insulin resistance that increases the risk of developing gestational diabetes.

"Carnipure tartrate has clear benefits for pregnant women. It not only maintains normal L-carnitine levels but also decreases plasma free fatty acids, thus potentially decreasing the risk for developing insulin resistance,"said lead researcher Prof. Alfred Lohninger from the Medical University of Vienna.

Established ingredient

L-carnitine occurs naturally in the human body and is essential for turning fat into energy. It is frequently used as a dietary supplement by physically active people to help with post-exercise recovery.

Lonza, which claims to be the world's largest manufacturer of L-Carnitine, has said that extensive scientific research shows the supplement promotes cardiovascular health and that other studies suggest the nutrient may be useful in weight management.

In terms of pregnancy, it has already been shown that levels of carnitine decrease during pregnancy, while the reason is unknown. A study published in the European Journal of Clinical Nutrition, suggested that this may be due to a decrease in the rate of carnitine biosynthesis, which may be due to an inadequate iron status in the women (Vol. 63, pp. 1098-1105).

Study details

Prof. Lohninger and his co-workers recruited 30 pregnant women in the 20th week of gestation and divided them into two groups: One groups received the L-carnitine supplements (2 grams per day) until week 38 of pregnancy, while the other group received a placebo. Twenty non-pregnant women also received placebo to act as an additional control group.

Results showed that pregnant women who received the L-carnitine supplements exhibited significant increases in the expression of carnitine acyltransferase enzymes, which play a role in the oxidation of fatty acids in the mitochondria – low expression of these enzymes are associated with increased levels of free fatty acids.

Pregnant women in the placebo group however experienced increases in levels of free fatty acids.

"The present study showed that supplementation with 2 grams of L-carnitine per day resulted in a 5- to 10-fold increase in the relative mRNA levels of carnitine acyltransferases […], thus reaching values which were found in non-pregnant healthy adults," wrote the researchers.

Source: Gynäkologisch-geburtshilfliche Rundschau (Journal for Obstetrics and Gynecology) Volume 49, Pages 230-235, doi:10.1159/000301075

"Relationship between Carnitine, Fatty Acids and Insulin Resistance"

Authors: A. Lohninger, U. Radler, S. Jinniate, S. Lohninger, H. Karlic, S. Lechner, D. Mascher, A. Tammaa, H. Salzer, H.

Excellent foods for people with DM. Chia, an ancient food; Coconut oil; Hemp protein

http://nutiva.com/chia/

Kombucha helps people with diabetes (PWD)

http://www.kombuchahome.com/how-to-make-kombucha-tea.html

Avoid fluoride if you have diabetes or thyroid dis-orders.

Fluoride impacts thyroid health which in turn creates risk to people with diabetes and can promote it.

Decades ago doctors always looked at the connection between thyroid and DM, many think DM is a thyroid dis-order.

Magnesium for health with diabetes:

Mineral Deficiency Associated with Complications of Impaired Blood Sugar (magnesium)

2010 Jun 16. According to a new study, diabetes-related kidney disease is associated with a deficiency of a particular mineral. Diabetes, which affects 23.7 million Americans, is the leading cause of kidney failure in the United States. The American Diabetes Association reports that in 2005, 44 percent of new cases of kidney failure were due to diabetes. Research indicates that the risk of developing kidney disease can be reduced by improved control of blood sugar and blood pressure in diabetics. Symptoms of diabetic kidney disease include fluid retention, loss of sleep, poor appetite, upset stomach, difficulty concentrating and generalized weakness.

In this recently published study, investigators evaluated blood levels of copper and magnesium in subjects with diabetic nephropathy (kidney disease). The subjects included 40 patients with diabetic nephropathy and 40 healthy individuals to serve as the control group. In addition to blood levels of copper and magnesium, the subjects were also evaluated for fasting blood sugar; postprandial (after eating) blood sugar; hemoglobin A1c, a measurement of blood sugar control over the previous 3 months; and microalbumin, a measurement of kidney function.

The results showed that fasting blood sugar, postprandial blood sugar, hemoglobin A1c, and microalbumin levels were significantly higher in the subjects with diabetic nephropathy compared to the control group. The study also found that blood magnesium levels were significantly lower in the subjects with diabetic kidney disease, compared with the control group. The researchers did not find an association between copper levels and diabetic nephropathy.

The study authors stated, "The findings in the present study suggest that hypomagnesemia [low magnesium] may be linked with development of diabetic nephropathy."

Reference: Prabodh S, Prakash DS, Sudhakar G, Chowdary NV, Desai V, Shekhar R. Status of Copper and Magnesium Levels in Diabetic Nephropathy Cases: a Case-Control Study from South India. Biol Trace Elem Res.

Avoid magnsium oxide whenever possible, it does not offer the best absorption or benefit.

If you were interested in a very good magnesium supplement I offer one and many other beneficial supplements too.

Magnesium intake and incidence of metabolic syndrome among young adults.

He K, Liu K et al

Circulation. 2006 Apr 4;113(13):1675-82.Epub 2006 Mar 27.

Department of Preventive Medicine, Feinberg School of Medicine, Northwestern University, Chicago, IL 60611, USA.

BACKGROUND: Studies suggest that magnesium intake may be inversely related to risk of hypertension and type 2 diabetes mellitus and that higher intake of magnesium may decrease blood triglycerides and increase high-density lipoprotein (HDL) cholesterol levels.

METHODS AND RESULTS: We prospectively examined the relations between magnesium intake and incident metabolic syndrome and its components among 4637 Americans, aged 18 to 30 years, who were free from metabolic syndrome and diabetes at baseline.

Metabolic syndrome was diagnosed according to the National Cholesterol Education Program/Adult Treatment Panel III definition. Diet was assessed by an interviewer-administered quantitative food frequency questionnaire, and magnesium intake was derived from the nutrient database developed by the Minnesota Nutrition Coordinating Center.

During the 15 years of follow-up, 608 incident cases of the metabolic syndrome were identified.

Magnesium intake was inversely associated with incidence of metabolic syndrome after adjustment for major lifestyle and dietary variables and baseline status of each component of the metabolic syndrome. Compared with those in the lowest quartile of magnesium intake, multivariable-adjusted hazard ratio of metabolic syndrome for participants in the highest quartile was 0.69 (95% confidence interval [CI], 0.52 to 0.91; P for trend <0.01). The inverse associations were not materially modified by gender and race. Magnesium intake was also inversely related to individual component of the metabolic syndrome and fasting insulin levels.

CONCLUSIONS: Our findings suggest that young adults with higher magnesium intake have lower risk of development of metabolic syndrome.

What is metabolic syndrome?

Metabolic syndrome is one word that covers a whole range of diseases from obesity that affects over half the population of the United States, to high blood pressure, insulin resistance, diabetes and heart disease. Magnesium deficiency along with deficiency of other major and minor trace minerals and an extreme daily intake of sodium (salt) have a major role to play in the most prevalent diseases of our time. The RDA for magnesium, which stands at 400 mg, may be too low when added as a supplement to reverse the effects of metabolic syndrome. Perhaps 400 mg of magnesium twice a day for adults would be better starting point for a magnesium deficient person.

A cure for type 1 diabetes?

Both types of diabetes are currently presented as incurable by the medical establishment. Apparently, only alleviation of symptoms is possible. However, in the case of type 1diabetes, where the patient's pancreas produces insufficient insulin to control blood glucose levels, huge progress has been made in India. Most type 2 patients can benefit by changing their diet.

Type 1 (insulin dependent) diabetes

In conventional medicine, type 1 diabetes patients are prescribed a variety of glucose-lowering drugs, principally insulin, which keep them alive and suppress the symptoms, but do not cure the disease.

Researchers in Madras, India are addressing what they believe may be the major cause: malfunction in pancreatic beta cells. Double-blind studies [1] confirm that the therapy they have developed can cure up to 60% of patients by restoring proper beta cell function. The deciding factor appears to be whether the antigens which originally caused the auto-immune response which damaged the beta cells are still in the patient's body. Where they remain in the body a cure is less likely because they continue to trigger damaging immune system activity. Work on how to remove the antigens continues.

The therapy

A water-soluble extract of the leaves of Gymnema sylvestre (400 mg/day) was administered to 27 patients for 10-12 months with type 1 diabetes on insulin therapy. Insulin requirements came down.

Fasting blood glucose levels fell.

While serum lipids (fats and oils) returned to near normal levels, fasting blood glucose levels remained higher than in healthy people. The control group (people with type1 diabetes on insulin therapy only) showed no significant reduction in serum lipids, or fasting blood glucose levels.

Gymnema sylvestre therapy appeared to enhance the body's own production of insulin, possibly by regeneration/revitalisation of the residual beta cells.

Whether the medical establishments in more industrially developed countries will allow the adoption of this herb-based therapy for diabetes is another matter.

Ed.- We recommend that people wishing to try Gymnema sylvestre do so in conjunction with a medical nutritionist. A fuller description of the therapy used in the type 1 diabetes trial is available free of charge from the Green Health Watch office (please send a stamped addressed envelope).

http://www.greenhealthwatch.com/newsstories/newsillnesses/cure-diabetes1.html

[1] Shanmugasundaram,ERB et al. Journal of Ethnopharmacology 1990;30:265-79 and 281-94

(11128) Thomas Smith. Nexus Magazine

The prevention and treatment of adult onset diabetes includes:

1. Protein: wild salmon, free range chicken and free range beef or lamb.

2. Complex carbohydrates (whole grains, legumes, and vegetables).

3. The avoidance of simple sugars and white flour.

4. Stevia, from the leaves of a plant that grows in South America; Just Like Sugar™, and are the best sweeteners to use. None of them affect blood glucose so they are safe to use in diabetes. Avoid Truvia as it has erythritol a sugar alcohol
http://naturalhealthnews.blogspot.com/2008/12/problems-with-new-sweetener.html

5. Don't use the sugar substitute, aspartame, which can worsen blood sugar control and cause weight gain, headaches, nerve damage, and eye damage, because it is made partly from wood alcohol, which breaks down to formaldehyde.

6. Emphasize fiber from oat bran, flaxseed, psyillium husk (NOT METAMUCIL because it has aspartame) and apples which all have a positive effect on keeping blood sugar balanced.

Read The Yeast Connection and Women's Health (Crook & Dean, 2005) and IBS for Dummies (Dean & Wheeler, 2005). Yeast can be cured naturally.

I also suggest that you try to identify possible allergies by eliminating likely suspects (dairy, wheat, corn) from the diet for several days and then eating several meals of one of the suspected foods in one day and see how you feel. Better yet do a blood test or finger stick for glucose levels. If your blood sugar is elevated after eating a particular food, avoid it.

Aspartame and Splenda

Web sites: www.mpwhi.com, www.dorway.com, www.wnho.net

Aspartame Toxicity Center, www.holisticmed.com/aspartame

A DIFFERENT LOOK AT SOLVING THE PROBLEM OF DIABETES TYPE 1

By Gayle Eversole CHI copyright 2000

Having been educated in depth in the scientific method at a time when it had place and meaning, I well understand the standard approach used daily in efforts to solve major health problems.

Combining my scientific, medical and natural medicine backgrounds and my natural bent to look at the world from different vectors, I am pleased to submit my approach to resolution of Diabetes 1.

1. Change requirements for Hepatitis B vaccines to infants and small children as it is clearly established that this vaccine is associated with the development of diabetes 1.

2. Utilize the following nutritional supplements which have been shown to effectively reduce the problem of diabetes 1: Zinc; 2: Vitamin D3.

3. Block use of artificial sweeteners, artificial flavors and colors in foods because these substances are documented to be associated with inflammation and in many cases diabetes. Adequate nutrition is the key to preventing most health problems, especially when supplements with vitamins and minerals.

4. Supplement with the herbal supplements (liquid extract form) 1: Marshmallow Root (for anti inflammation; 2: Astragalus (for deep immune enhancement)

5. Supplement with live cultures of acidophilus and bifidus to enhance gut and small intestine flora and protect the pancreas.

As we can openly move from the drug only approach to the many global health concerns there will be change.

Excellent Nutrition Website http://whfoods.org/

Can You Block Aging With a B-Vitamin?

Health News - By VRP Staff

Scientists may not be able to stop aging—but they do know one of the factors that causes many of the damaging effects of aging. Diabetes, inflammatory diseases, atherosclerosis, macular degeneration, arthritis, Alzheimer's disease, poor bone healing, cataracts and kidney disease... all of these common pathologies have been directly linked to advanced glycation end-products (AGEs), toxic molecules that are formed through a series of abnormal reactions between sugar, proteins and lipids.1-11

These AGEs accumulate slowly and silently in your body over time, where they serve to make your tissues stiffer and less elastic. In short: They age you, plain and simple.

Diabetes is probably the best example of the hidden dangers of AGE accumulation: Research shows that diabetics suffer from conditions like heart disease, kidney disease and nerve damage a full 20 to 40 years earlier than their healthy counterparts—while animal studies indicate that strategies aimed at inhibiting AGE production may reduce some of the disastrous effects AGEs have on the heart, kidney and nerves.12-13 But even if you're healthy, blocking AGEs can play a critical role in the preservation of your health... helping to slow your body's aging process in a manner similar to caloric restriction.

So how can you get the edge against AGEs—and start slowing down your own body's clock?

Surprisingly, the solution is easier than you might think.

In the last decade, scientists have discovered that benfotiamine—a synthetic, fat-soluble form of thiamine, or vitamin B1—is a potent AGE blocker. In fact, clinical studies show that this form of the vitamin is as much as 430 percent more bioavailable than its water-soluble counterparts, which have a modest absorption rate of only four to six percent.14-16

This superior absorption rate offers one reason for the powerful protection benfotiamine offers against AGEs—a benefit that's been borne out in a number of animal and human studies. In one study, for example, researchers found that type 1 diabetics given 600 mg of benfotiamine daily experienced a 40 to 69 percent drop in levels of carboxymethyllysine (CML) and methylglyoxal-derived AGEs—two predominant AGEs implicated in impaired cognitive and heart health and blood vessel complications within just four weeks.17

Additional trials have shown that supplementing with benfotiamine can also significantly support nerve health, while helping to regulate heartbeat and improve nerve conduction.18-19 And finally, animal studies suggest that benfotiamine supports eye health in diabetics, too.

In a 36-week study of three groups of rats—two of which were diabetic or hyperglycemic, along with one set of healthy controls—researchers found that rats receiving benfotiamine had retinas as healthy as controls by the end of the study. Those diabetic rats that did not receive benfotiamine, however, suffered severely damaged rentinal blood vessels as a result.20

To achieve the same level of scientifically supported AGE protection at home, get your daily dose of benfotiamine in capsule form.

Statins Increase Risk of Diabetes

These drugs also are a cause of peripheral neuropathy. You can safely lower cholesterol with natural products and actually triglycerides are a greater risk. They can be lowered too naturally.

http://naturalhealthnews.blogspot.com/2008/12/oh-i-know-you-are-one-of-those-health.html

www.medscape.com

From Medscape Diabetes & Endocrinology > Viewpoints

Do Statins Raise the Risk for Diabetes?

Gregory A. Nichols, PhD

Posted: 05/04/2010

Statins and Risk of Incident Diabetes: A Collaborative Meta-analysis of Randomised Statin Trials

Sattar N, Preiss D, Murray HM, et al

Lancet. 2010;375:735-742. Epub 2010 Feb 16.

Study Summary: Using data from 13 clinical trials with 91,140 participants, the investigators conducted a meta-analysis to determine whether a relationship exists between statin use and the development of diabetes. Six of the trials had previously published data for incident diabetes. The other 7 studies had not analyzed or published data on incident diabetes.

For each trial in the meta-analysis, odds ratios and 95% confidence intervals were calculated on the basis of the number of patients who did not have diabetes at baseline and the number who developed incident diabetes. An overall odds ratio was then calculated with a random-effects model meta-analysis. Meta-regression analysis was also used to investigate potential differences (heterogeneity) between trials. Specifically, baseline age, body mass index (BMI), and percentage of change in low-density lipoprotein (LDL) cholesterol were tested.

Of the 91,140 participants without diabetes, 4278 developed incident diabetes over a mean study follow-up of about 4 years. The rate of diabetes in individual trials varied substantially. Of the 13 trials, 2 independently showed positive associations between statin therapy and incident diabetes. In the combined data, 174 more cases of incident diabetes occurred in the groups assigned to statin treatment than in the placebo or standard-care groups, representing a 9% increase in the likelihood of development of diabetes during follow-up. The investigators estimated that this amounted to 1 additional case of diabetes per 255 patients treated with statins over 4 years. The results were nearly identical when the analyses were restricted to placebo-controlled trials. Heterogeneity between trials was low. Although the association between statin therapy and risk for incident diabetes was stronger in trials with older participants, baseline BMI and percent change in LDL cholesterol did not seem to be important factors.

Viewpoint - Although most statin trials to date had not found a relationship between statin use and diabetes incidence, the recent JUPITER (Crestor 20mg Versus Placebo in Prevention of Cardiovascular (CV) Events)[1] trial that reported an increased risk for diabetes in patients assigned to the rosuvastatin arm seconded concerns raised several years ago when the PROSPER (PROspective Study of Pravastatin in the Elderly at Risk)[2] trial reported similar findings with pravastatin. However, most trials had not looked at diabetes as a secondary outcome. The investigators of the current study are to be commended for obtaining access to previously unpublished results, thus eliminating a common flaw in meta-analyses.

With these data, they were able to identify a small but significantly increased risk for incident diabetes associated with statin use. Like observational studies, however, a meta-analysis cannot establish causation; therefore, it is possible that unmeasured factors explain the results. For example, the analysis did not account for baseline glycemic level. This is unlikely to be different between groups in randomized trials, but it is possible or even likely that patients who developed diabetes were more dysglycemic, and that a small "nudge" from statins was enough for them to convert to diabetes. If so, these patients were already at increased cardiovascular risk,[3] in which case treatment with statins would be far more important than the few milligrams per deciliter of fasting glucose that took these patients over the diagnostic threshold for diabetes. It is also important to note that these results do not address whether statins raise blood sugar in people already diagnosed with diabetes, most of whom should already be taking statins.[4]

References :

Ridker PM, Danielson E, Fonseca FA, et al; JUPITER Study Group. **Rosuvastatin to prevent vascular events in men and women with elevated C-reactive protein**. N Engl J Med. 2008;359:2195- 2207. AbstractShepherd J, Blauw GJ, Murphy MB, et al; PROSPER Study Group, PROspective Study of Pravastatin in the Elderly at Risk. Pravastatin in elderly individuals at risk of vascular disease (PROSPER): a randomised controlled trial. Lancet. 2002;360:1623-1630. Abstract Levitan EB, Song Y, Ford ES, Liu S.

Is nondiabetic hyperglycemia a risk factor for cardiovascular disease? A meta-analysis of prospective studies. Arch Intern Med. 2004;164:2147-2155. Abstract American Diabetes Association. Standards of Medical Care in Diabetes -- 2010. Diabetes Care. 2010;33(suppl1):S11-S61.

Authors and Disclosures - Author: Gregory A. Nichols, PhD

Investigator, Kaiser Permanente Center for Health Research, Portland, Oregon

Disclosure: Gregory A. Nichols, PhD, has disclosed the following relevant financial relationships: Received grants for clinical research from GlaxoSmithKline; Merck & Co., Inc.; Novartis Pharmaceuticals Corporation; Novo Nordisk

Medscape Diabetes & Endocrinology © 2010 WebMD, LLC

The brown rice and sesame seed blend as a breakfast food can do a great help to bring blood sugar levels to normal value.

From my blog - http://bit.ly/cgSnHC

http://naturalhealthnews.blogspot.com/2010/06/brown-rice-more-than-low-gl-or-high.html

This is an old approach for people with diabetes.

Why Vitamin C can reverse diabetes

The Endocrine Society's 92nd Annual Meeting held in San Diego was the site of a presentation on June 21, 2010 of the findings of a study involving adults with metabolic syndrome which found an improvement in insulin resistance among participants who received a diet enriched with antioxidant nutrients.

Metabolic syndrome is a cluster of risk factors that includes increases in waist circumference, blood pressure, fasting glucose and triglycerides, and a reduction in high density lipoprotein (HDL) cholesterol. Individuals with three or more of these conditions have a reduced ability to utilize insulin, and are at an increased risk of developing cardiovascular disease and diabetes. "Oxidative stress could play an important role in metabolic syndrome-related manifestations contributing to insulin resistance," write endocrinology researcher Antonio Mancini, MD and his associates at Rome's Catholic University of the Sacred Heart in the abstract summarizing their research. "The reciprocal influences between oxidative stress and insulin resistance are not clear."

The study included 16 men and 13 women aged 18 to 66 years with insulin resistance and obesity. All participants received a diet that provided 1,500 calories per day for three months. Half of the participants' diets contained fruits and vegetables that provide high amounts of antioxidant nutrients. The subjects were further divided into groups that received or did not receive 1000 milligrams per day of the drug metformin, which improves insulin sensitivity in patients with type 2 diabetes. Body mass index, glucose tolerance and other factors were assessed at the beginning and end of the study.

While all participants experienced similar decreases in body mass index, only those that received the antioxidant-enriched diet had significant reductions in insulin resistance, with the greatest benefits observed in those who also received Metformin.

The ability of antioxidants to help reduce oxidative stress may help protect against a number of conditions, including metabolic syndrome. "The beneficial effects of antioxidants are known, but we have revealed for the first time one of their biological bases of action—improving hormonal action in obese subjects with the metabolic syndrome," Dr Mancini stated.

Many of the vitamins like Vitamin B advanced, Thiamine or Vitamin B1 and Pyridoxine or Vitamin B6 are a great controller of diabetes.

Other vitamins like vitamin C and vitamin E conjointly work great in controlling diabetes. Take a look on the advantages how they will facilitate your controlling your diabetes

Vitamin C – Vitamin C is taken into account highly useful in treating diabetes. As a result of of stress, urinary losses and destruction by artificial sweeteners, the vitamin C requirement is sometimes high in diabetics. Massive amounts of this vitamin generally bring terribly sensible results. Dr. George V Mann in Perspective in Biology and Medication suggested additional vitamin C for diabetics. Natural insulin output increases in diabetics with supplementary doses of vitamin C The intake of vitamin C in the form of dried Indian gooseberry (amla), the richest known supply of vitamin C, or tablets of five hundred mg or from natural sources of vitamin C besides amla, are citrus fruits, green leafy vegetables, sprouted Bengal gram and inexperienced grams

Vitamin E – This vitamin reduces considerably the devastating vascular damage accompanying diabetes. Dr. Willard Shute in The Complete Book of Vitamins recommends 800-1600 IU of vitamin E daily to forestall arterial degeneration in diabetes. The high dose will prevent neuropathy, do not use soy based vitamin E.

A Swedish study also supports vitamin E therapy for treating diabetes. Vitamin E helps diabetics decrease their insulin requirements. It might be advisable for a diabetes patient to require a daily dose of two hundred IU of this vitamin for a fortnight at a time.

Wealthy Sources of Vitamin E. Valuable natural foods sources of this vitamin are wheat or cereal germ, whole grain products, fruits and inexperienced leafy vegetables, milk and all whole raw or sprouted seeds.

Different made sources of vitamin E are cold pressed crude vegetable oils, especially sunflower seeds, safflower, raw and sprouted seeds and grains, alfalfa, lettuce, almond, human milk etc.

Self treatment scheme for Diabetes (Ayurveda) (Homeopathy)

http://bashirmahmudellias.blogspot.com/2010/08/diabetes-can-never-be-curedwithout_02.html>

Diabetes and its miraculous medicines

Dear all,

Take these nine homeopathic medicines (as a cure for diabetes) according to my direction. I am optimistic that my formula will give a full cure for 95% of diabetic patients. Although few cases will not get full cure, still they will get tenfold better result than any other healing systems.

Take these medicines repeatedly in a cyclical way (i.e. after 0.- 9 start again from no.- 1). You can double the dose (i.e. 20 drops) if your sugar level is much higher. Yea, it is better to take all homeopathic medicines in empty stomach ; but you can take them after meal if you forget.

You should reduce other diabetic medicines to half after two weeks and totally stop all those rubbish medicines after four weeks. Try to buy Germany or U.S.A. made medicines. You can exclude any one of these nine medicines if it seems don't helping or causing serious side effects.

Do not change my recommendation on potency and dose, but you can take the nearest potency if the recommended potency is not available in the local market. In some rare cases, you may need to consult a homeopathic specialist to be able to use more precisely selected medicines (which best suit with your physical and mental make-up). When you are free from diabetes, then don't stop these medicines suddenly. Rather you should gradually decrease the dose (10 drops® 5 drops ® 2 drops) and in this way take three to six months to stop them totally. (N.B.- Must obey the diet rules & exercise.)

{Removing the causes of diabetes :- At the same time we need to remove the underlying cause of diabetes.

(1) If you got diabetes after a mental shock, you should take one dose (ie. one drop) of Natrum muriaticum 1M, then after one month of interval take one dose (ie. One drop) of Natrum muriaticum 10M and then after one month of interval take one dose (ie. One drop) of Natrum muriaticum 50M.

(2) If you got diabetes after vaccination, you should take one dose (ie. one drop) of Thuja occidentalis 1M, then again after one month of interval take one dose (ie. one drop) of Thuja occidentalis 10M and then after one month of interval take one dose (ie. one drop) of Thuja occidentalis 50M.

(3) If you have a family history of diabetes, you should take one dose (ie. one drop) of Syphilinum 1M, then after one month of interval take one dose (ie. one drop) of Syphilinum 10M and then again after one month of interval take one dose (ie. one drop) of Syphilinum 50M.

(4) If you have a family history of tuberculosis or Asthma or in the habit of catching cold frequently, you should take one dose (ie. One drop) of Bacillinum 1M, then after one month of interval take one dose

(ie. one drop) of Bacillinum 10M and then again after one month of interval take one dose (ie. one drop) of Bacillinum 50M.}

> (1) Acidum Phosphoricum Q - (Take this homeopathic medicine 10 drops 03 times daily for first week. mixing with half of a glass of water)

> (2) Gymnema sylvestra Q - (Take this homeopathic medicine 10 drops 03 times daily for second week. mixing with half of a glass of water)

> (3) Senecio aureus Q - (Take this homeopathic medicine 10 drops 03 times daily for third week. Mixing with half of a glass of water)

> (4) Calcarea Carbonica 30 - (Take this homeopathic medicine 10 drops 03 times daily for fourth week. mixing with half of a glass of water)

> (5) Syzygium Jambos Q - (Take this homeopathic medicine 10 drops 03 times daily for fifth week. mixing with half of a glass of water)

> (6) Arsenicum Bromatum Q - (Take this homeopathic medicine 10 drops 03 times daily for sixth week. mixing with half of a glass of water)

> (7) Iodium 30 - (Take this homeopathic medicine 10 drops 03 times daily for seventh week. mixing with half of a glass of water)

> (8) Acidum Picricum Q - (Take this homeopathic medicine 10 drops morning and afternoon for eighth week. mixing with half of a glass of water)

> (9) Sanicula Q - (Take this homeopathic medicine 10 drops 03 times daily for ninth week. mixing with half of a glass of water)

Dr. Bashir Mahmud Ellias

Author, Design specialist, Islamic researcher, Homeo consultant chamber: Jagarani homeo hall 47/4 Toyenabi circular road, (near ittefaq crossing & studio 27) Motijheel, Dhaka, Bangladesh.

Mob : +880-01916038527

E-mail : Bashirmahmudellias@hotmail.com

Website : http://bashirmahmudellias.blogspot.com

Thankfully access to Avandia has been limited since this was first reported. (2011)

First of all the cardiovascular risk of Avandia has been reported since 2004 and I do not believe it is a safe drug.

Avandia WILL increase cholesterol levels.

LOW THYROID WILL increase cholesterol levels.

More reasons why not to take statin drugs.

More about Avandia

http://www.patrickholford.com/index.php/blog/blogarticle/817/ Patrick is a colleague in the UK

http://www.bbc.co.uk/news/health-11170878

From my web site and related sources: www.leaflady.org:

http://www.leaflady.org/natural_healing_for_diabetes.htm Based on the course I used to offer in the 90s, taught at many reservations.

Aspartame Awareness weekend, 9/9-12
http://www.rense.com/general92/aspar.htm

Some Splenda info
http://naturalhealthnews.blogspot.com/2010/05/splenda-sucralose-what-itdoes. html

Increases A1C and more...Splenda

http://naturalhealthnews.blogspot.com/2010/05/cod-liver-oil-helps-prevent-diabetes.html

What women don't know about bone health can hurt them ...

For years you have heard how important it is to take hormone replacement therapy (HRT) in menopause to protect you from bone loss, but recent research has shown that this may in fact not be accurate, as bone health is dependent on many things.

• The work of Susan Love, MD supports the concept of not replacing something that is not supposed to be there.

• John Lee, MD has shown benefits with progesterone supplementation.

• The work of Susan Brown, a medical anthropologist at Syracuse University Medical School, has established the importance of a broad base of nutrients and dietary factors to insure bone health.

• Hormone Heresy, the work of Sherill Sellman, exposes much of the invalid information foisted upon women by the medical establishment.

Herbalists are doing fine work with women in an effort to teach them about the healing benefits of Red Raspberry Leaf, Red Clover, Sage, Chaste Tree Berry, and other herbs to protect bones.

What you may not have heard or read about is that Vitamin K, when given to post menopausal women, inhibits precipitous calcium loss, thereby protecting them from osteoporosis. Vitamin K is so effective that it can restore bone to premenopausal densities. Vitamin K, a fat soluble vitamin, is manufactured in your body in the large intestine or colon. In the large intestine naturally occurring "healthy" bacteria synthesize vitamins K and B. This is another reason to maintain a healthy colon.

Wholesome organic food will give you many choices for supplementing vitamin K in your diet. You can find Vitamin K in foods such as: cabbage, cauliflower, soybeans, whole grains, wheat germ, wheat bran, potatoes, tomatoes, dark green leafy vegetables like spinach and kale, alfalfa, corn, mushrooms, oats, peas, and strawberries.

One hundred grams of the following sampling of foods, raw unless noted, contain the listed amounts of vitamin K in milligrams (mg.): quinoa 740 mg; adzuki beans 532 mg; peanuts 732 mg; tempeh 367 mg; pistachio nuts 1093 mg; pumpkin seeds 807 mg; almonds 732 mg; avocado 599 mg; dates 652 mg; figs 712 mg; raisins 746 mg; beet greens 909 mg; lima beans 570 mg; dandelion leaves 397 mg; garlic 401 mg; ginger root 415 mg; kale 447 mg; parsley 536 mg; spinach 558 mg; winter squash 437 mg; baked yam 816 mg; lightly steamed or poached halibut 576 mg, and rainbow trout 634 mg.

© Gayle Eversole, CRNP, PhD, AHG - 13 January, 2000

Vitamin K for better absorption of nutrients

Important in dental and gum problems; spider veins on face or legs; osteoporosis; and health concerns where nutrient absorption is in question! The American Journal Clinical Nutrition Jan 1999 gave results of a study of 72,000 nurses who were followed for 10 years evaluated dietary intake and the rate of hip fractures. The results were that the women whose diet included more Vitamin K were more protected from hip fractures. Homeopathic Vitamin K can help with absorption of Vitamin K from foods such as green vegetables-lettuce, green beans, fermented soy foods, whole grains.

In an article published in the January, 2009 issue of The Journal of Pediatrics, researchers at Boston's Joslin Diabetes Center report that 76 percent of diabetic teens examined had inadequate levels of vitamin D. Insufficient vitamin D levels in childhood prevents the attainment of optimal bone mass, and can increase fracture risk later in life.

Lori M. B. Laffel, MD, MPH, who is Chief of the Pediatric, Adolescent and Young Adult Section at Joslin, along with colleagues from Children's Hospital in Boston, measured serum 25-hydroxyvitamin D levels in 128 diabetic boys and girls aged 1.5 to 17.5 years. Participants included those with recent onset of type 1 diabetes as well as those with long-established disease.

While 24 percent of the youths had sufficient vitamin D levels, 61 percent were classified as insufficient and 15 percent as deficient. Deficiency tended to occur in older subjects, with only 15 percent of adolescents demonstrating vitamin D adequacy.

"To our surprise, we found extremely high rates of vitamin D inadequacy," stated Dr Laffel. "We didn't expect to find that only 24 percent of the study population would have adequate levels."

"We need to make sure all youths in general are getting enough vitamin D in their diets," commented lead author Britta Svoren, MD, who is a member of Joslin's Pediatric, Adolescent and Young Adult Section and the Section on Genetics and Epidemiology. "And, we need to pay particular attention to those with diabetes as they appear to be at an even higher risk of vitamin D deficiency. For children who are not drinking sufficient amounts of vitamin D fortified milk, we are encouraging them to take a vitamin D supplement of 400 IU daily. Many cereals are fortified with vitamin D as well."

An article published in the November, 2008 issue of Diabetes Care revealed an association between improved insulin resistance and vitamin K supplementation in men. Resistance to the effects of insulin characterizes type 2 diabetes, and can also occur among those at risk of developing the disease.

In a randomized, double blinded trial, researchers from Tufts University in Boston administered 500 micrograms vitamin K1 or a placebo daily for three years to 142 men and 213 women without diabetes. Plasma insulin, glucose and vitamin K1 levels, insulin resistance were assessed before the trial and at 6 and 36 months.

Although there was no association between vitamin K and insulin levels or insulin resistance observed in women by the end of the study, men who received the vitamin experienced a significant reduction in both. The authors suggest that the discrepancy between men and women to may be due to the increase in body fat that occurred among the women over the course of the three years, which may enhance storage of the fat-soluble vitamin, rendering it unavailable for peripheral organs. In the current study, women who had a greater body mass index were found to have lower levels of plasma vitamin K.

The authors propose that vitamin K could improve insulin sensitivity by suppressing inflammation.

Vitamin K has been shown to lower induced inflammation in both cell culture and animal studies.

Additionally, a recent observational study revealed a reduction in inflammatory markers associated with increased measures of vitamin K status.

The authors concluded that "Vitamin K supplementation for 36 months at doses attainable in the diet may reduce progression of insulin resistance in older men.

DISCLAIMER: *Any health related information in this publication is for educational purposes only. None of the information is to be construed as medical advice. Before applying any therapy or use of herbs, you may want to seek advice from your health care professional. This information should not be interpreted as a substitute for physician evaluation or treatment by a health care professional, and is not intended to provide or confirm a diagnosis.*

Gayle Eversole

CREATING HEALTH INSTITUTE

CHI began in 1988. We were certified as a 501c3 non-profit, tax-exempt organization early in 1989. Our focus is education about natural health and public health. We serve those with limited access to natural health, Elders, and people on reservations, as well as anyone interested in our services or products. All profits go to programs. Donations are welcome to help us continue this important work.

CHI – Creating Health Institute

Celebrating 50+ years, blending science with the natural healing arts.

*herbal*YODA Says! is a public service and part of the long established Health Matters© series from CHI.

TOC manages all educational services, publications and this newsletter. We're read around the world by thousands daily; please share our newsletter with your friends. This newsletter is written by Gayle Eversole, DHom, PhD, MH, NP, ND, founder and director of Creating Health Institute (CHI) and The

The Oake Centre for natural health education (TOC).

CHI is a tax-exempt, non-profit 501(c) (3) organization since 1989. We ask that you consider helping us continue this important work through your tax-deductible donations, and through purchases of our goods and services. Donating directly via PayPal (membership not required), and searching the web or doing your on-line shopping at www.goodsearch.com in support of Creating Health Institute helps us continue this important work.

"Frequently Copied, Never Duplicated!"

May the Creator of all mercies

scatter light

and not darkness

on our path.

ABOUT THE AUTHOR

Gayle Eversole, DHom, PhD, MH, NP, ND, has been studying and using natural healing for more than 50 years. She received her nursing degree from Neumann College in Aston, PA, and is a member of Sigma Theta Tau, national honor society for nursing there. She has worked for more than thirty five years in the medical profession as a nurse practitioner, consultant, administrator and educator. She serves on the medical advisory board of several health organizations and has worked in health care planning. Dr. Eversole offers legal and forensic nursing and mediation /arbitration for health concerns and Indian health issues, and is a widely respected health coach. She serves as a consultant to nutrition and herbal product companies, hosts a radio program, publishes a natural health eZINE, and maintains a clinical practice specializing in complex and complicated health problems. She is the author of My Happy Garden and My Medicine Garden and contributes to many books and articles on natural health care. Dr. Eversole continues to do research in natural health care, enjoys public speaking and writing articles in this field.

She has two grown daughters, one an artist working in the healing arts and one working in public relations.

Dr. Eversole offers classes to health care professionals, members of the public, business, organizations and government agencies.

For more information please see Health Forensics, www.healthforensics.org.

www.ingramcontent.com/pod-product-compliance
Lightning Source LLC
Chambersburg PA
CBHW022249290526
45785CB00015B/408